"If skincare has always been a mystery to you, this book will help you understand just how to bring your skin to a healthy glow easily and naturally."
- Shannon O'Brien
  Licensed Esthetician, Sugar Expert, AKA "The Sugar Mama,"
  The Dean of iSugarUniversity.com and creator of The Sugar Show

"This is a must-read book for every woman who wants to achieve healthy & beautiful skin through healthy, non-toxic solutions."
- Abbie Major
  Licensed Esthetician and owner of Abbie Major, Skin Love

"For women of all ages, this book simply and elegantly explains how to achieve beautiful, healthy, ageless skin. Everything you need to know is right here."
- Jeffrie Ann Chambers
  Licensed Esthetician and owner of Jeffrie Ann Chambers
  Skin Care

"Thought provocative and engaging, this book is what every woman needs to rediscover her beautiful skin from the inside out."
- Jackie Camacho-Ruiz
  Founder & Director of JJR Marketing,
  Keynote Speaker and Author of 8 books, including
  The Little Book of Business Secrets that Work!

skin deep

Demystifying Skin Care Solutions to Achieve Healthy, Glowing Skin

Samantha Dench

THE SKIN DISRUPTER

Fig Factor Media LLC

FIG
FACTOR
MEDIA

Edited by Cindy Tschosik of SoConnected LLC.
Cover Design and Layout by Carrie Keppner.

Printed and bound in the U.S.A.

ISBN # 978-0997160529

*I dedicate this book to my favorite angel
in heaven, Grandma Dotty.*

Dedication

As far back as I can remember, Dotty was always playing "witch doctor" and healing cuts with oils, honey or random items she had around the house. When we were sick, she always had a remedy to help us feel better. She also gave me my first "facial." Her old-school method began with a facial scrub, followed with holding my face above the steam with a towel over my head to "open up my pores." We then applied a peel-off mask from back in the day. We watched each other in the mirror to see who could peel it off in one piece. She won every time!

Dotty was more than my first skin care teacher. She was my second mother. Whenever I think about my childhood, I remember that she was always at my school events, dance recitals, graduations and all our family vacations.

She opened up her heart, and love
was the only thing that poured out of her.

Everyone was welcome in her home and her life. She hosted every holiday with love and passion and her motto was "Come Early, Stay Late." She was the greatest entertainer and always loved a good party. Anytime there was an excuse to celebrate, Dotty gave it 100% every time. She loved everyone and everyone loved her.

When I think about my greatest role model, it is Dotty. She was kind, loving and always had a smile on her face. If I could aspire to be one person, it would be her. When I think about love and support, my family was and is always by my side. Dotty was always my #1 cheerleader. She never tried to talk me out of anything and always encouraged me to follow my heart and give it my all.

She was there for me through all my poor choices and bad decisions, but she never judged me or showed anger or disappointment — a quality very few people possess. When I finally decided to become an esthetician, she was thrilled and she was my very first client. I'll never forget the day she passed. I realized that my favorite person was gone, and I realized how much I would miss her visits to my spa for facials, and how she praised me for my touch.

Dotty is a true angel in this world, and I know she would be so proud of me. I know that she was with me every step of the way while I was writing this book and every step of my crazy, life-changing move to Austin. Whenever I am sad, I think of Dotty and feel her with me. I just wish she was still here to read this book.

Thank you, Grandma Dotty, for teaching me how to keep my skin healthy, for always being there for me and for imprinting my heart and soul with your love.

I will love you forever.

Table of Contents

Preface

Samantha Dench... The Speaker

The Real Deal. That is how I would describe Samantha Dench. I heard her speak at an event in January, 2016. With her spa coat on, healthy glowing face and a pleasant smile, she spoke passionately and scientifically about caring for skin from the inside out. What? Hmmm. That is interesting.

At that time, I was having all sorts of problems. Being a rosacea sufferer, yes, I suffer. I've learned to not take pictures without makeup. Forget about change of seasons; dry, flaky patches, wet, crisp whatever you call it. It's not pretty. Desiring to forego prescriptions for healthier options, I had started using a home party skin care brand. After the first round, it was worse. The rep tried to help and recommended the line for sensitive skin. It still was not the product line for me. Within 6 weeks, my face looked like raw meat. I was hardly recognizable. It itched; it burned. I should have worn a bag over my face.

Samantha Dench... The Esthetician & Spa Owner

Enter Samantha. Her points on diet, hydration, products and ingredients spoke to me and made sense. Her approach from the science of skin was refreshing and interesting. I never thought of the skin as an organ, much less a 'self-healing' organ. I liked her healthy approach. I booked my first spa appointment, and it was the start of change. We went through my products, she performed the consultation and facial and made recommendations. It killed me to buy a new line because I had just spent so much money on 2 lines that didn't work.

I started the products, and saw results within 3 days. Less burning and a fresh, clean feeling. We went on for a few months. It was definitely better, but I still had some issues. Finally, I went to the dermatologist. He explained that I had a severe flare up, which was alarming because it was better than before! He prescribed the cleansing cloths, the gel, the antibiotic—all that I was trying to avoid when I switched to the party-line products. It cleared up in less than two weeks, and I returned to Samantha's product line. It worked! Once I reached a neutral level, I could get off the medicated program and use a healthier line. My skin has never looked so good.

Samantha Dench... The Author

Enter the book. It is slightly unusual that the editor of the book would write the preface, but given my experience over the year of Samantha treating my skin issues, getting to know her vast and impressive in-depth knowledge about the science of skin and absorbing her content has given me the privilege to provide an exemplary recommendation about her to you.

During my first facial, she shared her story. Every writer loves a story. And then she shared her dream to write a book. What?! I'm a ghostwriter. And so, it began. Our first meeting was to discover the order and strategy. She came prepared with years of content in print, in video, and in her mind. If they could, they would give her a skin science award. She is extremely knowledgeable and smart about all things skin related. In addition to her knowledge, she has the gifted ability to clearly explain it to others. Our journey to make her dream come true began.

While you read this book, you will learn everything you need to know and more to meet your skin care goals. Samantha eloquently teaches how the skin can heal itself, how various products and ingredients help or hinder healthy skin, and how your skin care regimen can help you achieve your goals. Furthermore, how various diets, spa services and estheticians can heal skin issues and / or promote your healthy glow. In addition to her goal to educate you, she entwines fun anecdotes and stories along the way, which makes it not only a comprehensive guide that you will find valuable, intriguing and enlightening, but fun to read, as well.

It has been an honor to get to know Samantha both professionally and personally, and I am grateful to her for the many attributes she amplifies in her business: honesty, work ethic, compassion, sincerity about her care for each client, dedication to the science of the skin and industry news, and her passion to share it with all of us, so we can be healthy on the inside and out. May you find yourself "Skin Deep" in a fabulous read!

To Your Health,
Cindy Tschosik
Samantha's Client & Editor

Acknowledgements

Thank you, Evan, for standing by my side and taking care of the kids while I spent countless hours in the 5am club, weekends and nights writing this book.

To my kids, Zachary, Jonah, and Zoe, who love to hear me talk about this book. Thank you for your sheer excitement in this journey with me and for your watchfulness to see this book journey happen. Zachary, I promise you will get my computer very soon.

Thank you to my mom and dad who have always been supportive of EVERY job or next best thing that I wanted to do. You never stopped encouraging me to seek the next thing that spoke to my soul. Without you, I would never have kept going until I found it. You have always believed in me, and you still believe in me. You are my lead cheerleaders and greatest support system. You are my role models and dear friends. I cannot express how grateful I am to you both. Thank you for your support and help so I could achieve this lifelong dream. I love you both from the bottom of my heart.

I am truly grateful to have a family who always taught me to follow my dream. Throughout my childhood, my parents owned their own businesses, which led me to become an entrepreneur. My mom encouraged me to start my skin care business, and she taught me that

I can be a working mom and still be home for my kids. My dad is my rock, and he will always stand by me and support everything I do with love.

Thank you to my two BFF's, my sisters Sabrina and Salena, who are both inspiring women, sisters, friends and business owners who will always be here for me no matter what.

I am grateful to my grandparents who always supported me in everything I ever did. Together, they were the most loving, caring and amazing second parents to us three girls. They welcomed us into the world with loving arms and never once judged or complained.

I have to give another HUGE THANK YOU to Lori Crete and Pamela Vendetti for changing my life and for giving me the confidence I needed personally and professionally. This book never would have happened had I not taken that scary step to invest in business coaching. Thank you, both, for all the profound guidance you provide estheticians. When I started this book, I was in a completely different place. Over the last year, all the changes I was searching for came into my life at the exact time I needed them.

Thank you to my dear friend, Joy Klein, who under her guidance, told me this book needed to get written ASAP! Then right after that, the people who helped me on my journey showed up, guided me and shaped this book to be exactly what it is.

Thank you, Cindy Tschosik, for taking my ideas, notes, videos and putting them in order. Then once it was written, for taking my jumbled writings and re-writing and re-structuring this book to shape it into the masterpiece it is today. I may have written the book, but you made it sound amazing.

And if anyone would like skin care advice, Cindy is my official Esthetician Assistant because the knowledge she learned by living and breathing this book for so many months has given her a knowledge about skin that she never knew.

Thank you, Jackie Camacho-Ruiz, for guiding me through the beginning steps and for seeing the visions for this book's future. You are an inspiration to me. I am grateful for the privilege of working with you during the book publication process. Thank you for sharing all your secret tools and team of people you have available to help bring this to launch. You taught me how to create excitement as the publication process was happening which was so much fun!

Thank you, Carrie Keppner, for creating my brand and designing the cover and each interior page. You made it beautiful, and your love for this book is on every page that is read. You have such a beautiful gift and talent for design, and you show up as a professional every step of the way.

To my Book Team, I am truly grateful we met and look forward to books 2 & 3, as well as future projects. I wish you great success and hope only the best opportunities come your way from helping me with this book.

Thank you to my dear friends, Katt, Sarah, Kristen, Christal, Amy, Dawn, Perrin, Karen, Lindie, and Natalie for being here for me and supporting me in the most supportive and positive way. You are my tribe! I am blessed to have found the most fulfilling friendships in all of you and your never-ending support propels me forward every day.

Thank you, Tricia, for always sharing business & health tips with me. You are an incredible esthetician and friend. We are so alike and share the same passion for skin. I am so grateful to have you in my life!

I have been working very hard to grow as a person, mom, friend, professional and business owner. I made some decisions in my business and invested in a business coach who not only helped me in all areas of my life, but created a world for estheticians who are like-minded and WANT to do everything they can to help their clients.

They do it in a loving, caring way. Until now, I never knew this community existed; the friendships I've made from these groups and the amazing support I have received writing this book have changed my life in the most positive way.

I dedicate this book to my grandma, Dotty, who was my first skin care teacher, "the witch doctor," with her crazy natural healthy ways to heal the skin. The funny thing was they always worked! Honey on a bee sting or spoonfuls of honey to soothe a sore throat. If there was a cut, scrape, bruise or any sort of skin irritation, Dotty was there with a natural remedy and she always made it better. Maybe it was the ingredient, but I think it was her special touch. She had a way about her that was so calming and caring. Her touch is what healed more than the cut, she healed your heart. I miss Dotty. I wish she was still here today and could read this book because she would have been so proud, and she would have shared my book with the world!

As I reflect on my life, I am humbled, honored and grateful beyond measure to been blessed with women and men who surround me with such positive support and motivating encouragement. You all push me to want to do and be greater than I am at this moment. Through this project, I share your inspiration with the world, so they too, are supported, motivated and propelled to do and be greater.

I want to share that this journey of writing my book was more than I imagined. The opportunities offered were unexpected and delightful surprises. The friendships that have grown enrich me personally and professionally. The knowledge I've gained from writing the content of the book, especially the ingredient section, has expanded my view of the industry and reinforced my passion to help others in any way I can. Above all, the experience of working with a talented, dedicated and supportive team taught me that no matter how simple we find thoughts or words to be, they can be turned into a masterpiece when we open our hearts and let the masters guide us into the person we are to become.

Writing this book has given me more knowledge about the skin to help guide me as an esthetician, and it has helped me grow as a person. As a result, this book changed my life. I wrote the book while living in Illinois, but my heart pulled me to Austin, which was the craziest thing I've ever done in my life. I remember thinking a few years back how I wished I could shout out these words to the world and always tried to figure out how to make that happen. Now living on the opposite end of the country, I am finding my voice. I am finding that life always starts you on a journey and throws crazy turns in to see how you will respond. I have never been a big risk-taker, but after stepping up to a new adventure, I'm hooked. I can't wait to see what life throws at me with books 2 and 3!

I hope, from the bottom of my heart, that you enjoy reading this book as much as I enjoyed writing it. Take as much knowledge as you can, so you, too, can be educated and make the right choices for your own skin to look and feel beautiful from the inside out.

skin deep

Demystifying Skin Care
Solutions to Achieve Healthy,
Glowing Skin

Part 1: Above & Below the Skin

Introduction

Samantha's Story Time

My grandparents' house was my second home. My grandma, Dotty, and I would have our special time which included an 'at-home facial.' She would sit me over one of those face steamers to "open up my pores" with a towel over my head. We applied a peel-off mask to our faces. When it was time to remove it, we stood together in front of her mirror and watched to see who could peel it off in one piece. She won every time.

Looking back on my history, as I write this book, skin care was ingrained in me at an early age. When it came time to decide college and career, I was your typical 18-year old who had no clue what to be when I grew up. It took me until I was 23 before I decided to attend esthetics school. Before that, I loved to dance, so off I went for my first year of college as a dance major who, after a few months, realized that I did NOT have a dancer's body and would never be picked as a lead dancer. I barely finished out my first year and came home to rethink my life.

The second fall, I attended community college and again had no clue, so that didn't last long either. In 2000, I finally decided on web design and earned my Associate Degree in 2001. The problem: employers wanted 3-5 years of experience in web design. So I worked several odd jobs in offices, hoping that I would stumble upon the right job or right fit. I liked being in an office, but didn't like being confined all day except for the lunch break.

In 2003, my mom suggested that I go to school for makeup because I was a makeup junkie. I researched options and thought to myself, "What do I have to lose?" I signed up for school (once again).

Turns out, I HATE applying makeup to other people, BUT I fell in love with the science behind the skin. My career was born. I made it through 750 hours of esthetics school. I loved everything about facials and the fact that I could be a chemist to find the right ingredients and products to treat my clients. I finished at the top of my class, which was funny because I almost failed out of biology and chemistry in high school.

When estheticians leave esthetics school with their license, we are all smiley and excited to embark on our dream career. Our options are plentiful. We can work in day-spas, salons, or medical-spas for dermatologists. We are now even able to specialize in specific areas, such as medical, brow expert, waxing, a wellness-based approach and more. My opportunities included working 3 years for a med-spa and 2 for a day-spa.

After 5 years as an esthetician, I wanted to start a family. I really wanted to be home more than spa life would allow. In 2010, I decided to open my spa, Skin Deep, but I wanted to offer a different approach than my previous employers and local esthetic services, spas, or salons. During both positions, I learned a great deal about how the skin is affected by internal and external factors such as food, products, ingredients, and the environment.

They say timing is everything because just before my first pregnancy, I suffered a severe acne problem that ultimately flared up after each pregnancy over the next 7 years. With each pregnancy, my skin cleared up, so, like most women, I attributed it to hormones. But it wouldn't clear up after the births. At a previous position, my boss shared that some clients have too much yeast in their bodies.

Intrigued and driven to find understanding and answers, I began the quest to learn more about how the skin and internal organs are connected and how each is impacted by how we treat the skin. I voraciously read industry magazines, researched various services at the local spas and dug deep into the science of the skin to find a better understanding of how the interactions of food, products, ingredients and the environment play a significant role in skin issues. I changed my diet and healed myself from the inside. My acne disappeared!

I am NOT a dietician, nor do I have any background in nutrition. However, I am an avid researcher, and I have many industry colleagues, friends, and clients who share their success stories of the correlation between healthy living and skin improvement. Repeatedly, I have witnessed significant results with changes to diet, healthy choices, products, and ingredients. I love that this has not only helped my own skin clear up, but I'm helping change the lives of my clients too!

As Americans, we are shifting to incorporating alternative lifestyles to improve our health, skin and bodies in a natural way versus prescription medicine and medical doctors. I'm not saying doctors or medicine is bad. The medical field has made amazing strides in medicine, and doctors have impressive technology to treat and heal certain conditions. What I do believe is that action, education, information, healthy lifestyles, and consistent habits can prevent certain conditions.

After all the research, interviewing industry experts, and identifying my goals, my philosophy took root and dictated that my values and services were going to follow the healthiest approach to skin care.

At Skin Deep, we focus on healing from the inside out with healthy living, customized services and non-chemical products.

It took a year to finally find the right product line that aligned with my philosophy, values and services. I love that I am able to offer specialized services and custom products to help my clients reach their skin care goals, whether it is to clear up various skin issues and / or achieve a healthy glow.

As a licensed esthetician, it is my mission to teach each person how to prevent, protect and address skin issues with the healthiest and most productive approach possible. When I give a facial to my clients, I am not just working on the skin. I also identify what changes can be made on the inside to support healthier skin.

Along the way, this has truly been an amazing journey of learning and opening my eyes to opportunities for which I was not even aware. Writing this book helps me reach more people. It allows me to help you achieve your skin care goals, make healthy decisions and prevent skin issues. I really love to help you take better care of your skin, to live a healthier life and to love the skin you are in!

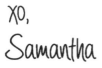

XO,
Samantha

Chapter 1:

Skin Anatomy

Did you know that the skin is the largest organ of the human body? It certainly is, and it is therefore connected to every organ in our body. *The skin has two layers called the epidermis and the dermis. The epidermis is the top layer of skin and is made up of dead skin cells. When we touch our skin, we touch the epidermis. The second layer is the dermis, which contains blood vessels, lymph vessels, hair follicles, and glands that produce sweat and oil.*[1] Want to know the skinny on our skin? Let the fun begin! Skin Anatomy 101 will cover the purpose and functions of the two main layers along with the sublayers of each.

THE EPIDERMIS LAYER

The epidermis has four layers with different functions to help the skin do its job.

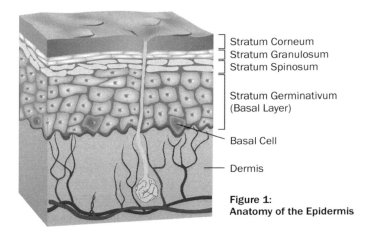

Stratum Corneum
Stratum Granulosum
Stratum Spinosum

Stratum Germinativum
(Basal Layer)

Basal Cell

Dermis

Figure 1:
Anatomy of the Epidermis

Stratum Germinativum (Basal Layer)

The stratum germinativum is better known as the "basal layer" which is the bottom layer of the epidermis. During the cell renewal process, new cells are formed. The new skin cells are pushed to the surface, die and eventually become the new surface of the epidermis. This process takes about 28 days for the full cycle. However, once we age, the process slows down and can require 45-60 days.

Throughout the process, new skin cells are called basal cells. Basal cells are constantly dividing to allow new cells to push their way to the skin's surface. The basal layer also contains cells called melanocytes. These melanocytes give skin its color by producing a pigment, called melanin. That gorgeous sun tan we all love is an increase in melanin pigment. Skin cells have a memory of their own and over many years, the melanocytes become damaged or their memory fades. This is important to remember because some melanocyte cells eventually under-produce or over-produce melanin, causing uneven skin tone, spots or dark patches.

Stratum Spinosum

The stratum spinosum is known as the spiny layer or prickle cell layer because as the basal cells move here, they begin to shrink and take on a spiky formation. The keratinization process begins, which means the nucleus and organelles disappear during this process. Metabolism ceases and the cells begin a programmed death as they become keratinized and rise to the stratum corneum.

Stratum Granulosum

The stratum granulosum is a very thin layer in the epidermis and functions by binding keratin. It is also known as the granular layer because the cells become granular as they reach the stratum granulosum. A fascinating fact to know about this layer is that the cells secrete lipids and proteins into the space between the cells as the cells begin to transition into the stratum corneum.

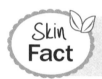

Skin Fact

The cells are the bricks and the lipids are the mortar acting as "glue" to hold the dead skin cells in place.

Stratum Corneum

The stratum corneum consists of 15-20 layers of dead skin cells, and it acts as the protective layer. It functions as a protector, producing dead skin cells to shield live cells from sun, environmental pollution and dirt. These dead skin cells are mostly keratin, which is a protein. Mixed in with the skin cells are lipids, which consist of ceramides, cholesterol and fatty acids. Think of this layer as bricks and mortar. The cells act as the bricks and the lipids acts as "glue" to hold the dead skin cells in place. The skin naturally exfoliates 1-2 layers of stratum corneum each day. The cells are microscopic and invisible to the eye. As the skin cells rise to the surface of our skin, they flatten and become fragments of the actual cell. During the process, the cells compress, causing them to lose their nucleus and cell organelles.

Stratum Lucidum

The stratum lucidum is a fifth layer of skin on the palms of the hands and the soles of the feet to provide heavier protection for our most used body parts. This thicker layer is found between the stratum corneum and the stratum granulosum layers.

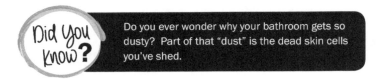

Did you know? Do you ever wonder why your bathroom gets so dusty? Part of that "dust" is the dead skin cells you've shed.

THE DERMIS LAYER

The dermis is the second layer of skin beneath the epidermis. This layer contains collagen, elastin and receptors that provide the sense of touch and temperature. It also contains hair follicles, sweat glands, oil glands, lymph vessels and blood vessels. The blood and lymph vessels are very important because they nourish the skin while also removing waste. The dermis contains two layers, papillary and reticular.

Papillary Dermis

The papillary dermis is named for its finger-like projections, called papillae, which contain the blood vessels. In addition, this layer contains hair follicles, receptors, sweat and oil glands.

Reticular Dermis

The reticular dermis is located beneath the papillary layer and contains the collagen and elastin fibers. These are protein-based fibers that are woven together to give the skin its strength and structure. The skin's pores reach down to the reticular dermal layer. Even though it is at the base of the skin, the reticular dermal layer accumulates damage from external pollution, environmental harm, sun damage and toxins or improper product use. Over time, collagen and elastin fibers begin to break down, causing fine lines and wrinkles. The fibers, which are like a net, stretch with our facial movement. After years of stretching this "net," the skin no longer returns to its original state.

The Subcutaneous Layer Inside the Body

There is one more layer beneath the dermal layer, which is called the subcutaneous layer. This layer is where the body stores fat, and it acts as a cushion for the skin. It is not considered a skin layer in the face area, but mostly for the body.

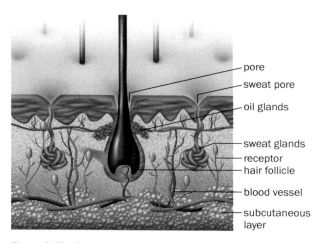

Figure 2: The Dermis Layer

Chapter 2:
How Products Penetrate the Skin

Our skin is an amazing organ! We don't think of our skin as a complex system, but as you read in the last chapter, there are a lot of functions our skin provides every day, even though it's as thin as a sheet of paper.

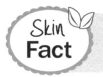

The skin is as thin as a sheet of paper, and the system is extremely complex with three layers and seven sublayers!

It may be surprising to learn that the skin is quite impenetrable, even for skin care products. The only time the skin can be penetrated is when the skin has been compromised with a cut or wound. Oftentimes, harsh treatments such as aggressive exfoliation treatments, improper products or injuries penetrate the skin, and leave openings for infection, skin damage and scarring. Under state regulations, estheticians are only allowed to work on the top layer of the skin, the stratum corneum of the epidermis. To care for the epidermis, estheticians use "product delivery systems" to cleanse, moisturize and treat the skin. The skin's pH level and quality of product helps decide the appropriate system.

Scientists have devoted many years of research to find the best solutions for skin care. They have developed many products and ingredients to penetrate the skin's barrier and reach the dermal level, the second main layer of skin. Actual products that penetrate the dermal layer include prescriptions, such as medical patches to curb smoking, induce birth control, reduce pain and deliver medicine.

Transdermal drug delivery is an exciting and challenging area. Currently, there are numerous dermal delivery systems on the market. However, the transdermal market is still limited to a narrow range of drugs. *Further advances in transdermal delivery depend on the ability to overcome the existing challenges faced regarding the permeation and skin irritation of the drug molecules.*[2]

When a patch is applied, the medicine is delivered through the skin into the blood stream. Unfortunately, some patients complain about irritation at the patch site because the skin is so delicate compared to the medication. It is always best to apply a patch to a different location each time. My sister had to wear a heart monitor patch during certain periods of the day and night. It was summer, and she wore tank tops. Her skin constantly itched and burned where the sun kissed the patch location. Fortunately, it didn't turn into a skin condition or illness, but it was very uncomfortable for her. Even without a "medicine delivery system," the skin can get irritated from patch material, which is typical. Patches are made of plastic or cloth materials. The plastic irritated my sister's skin. Cloth materials seem gentler.

Do you remember science class and the pH experiments that taught us that food can be acidic or alkaline? Our skin can be more acidic or alkaline, too. For the skin to absorb products and for delivery systems to function properly, skin needs to be at a neutral pH. A neutral pH for the skin is 4.5-5.5. Many factors can impact pH levels. For example, skin can become too acidic or too alkaline from using the wrong products. Too much alpha-hydroxy acids (AHA), beta-hydroxy acids (BHA) or retinols can cause the skin to have too many toxins. However, specially formulated products can help skin reach the appropriate level.

Since transdermal medications are carried through the bloodstream, they are not primarily used for skin care. However, there are several options for the product to penetrate the stratum corneum, also known as the first layer in the epidermis. Even though the skin is our protector, scientists are trying to break the barrier of medicinal penetration. Not all penetration is bad, as medicinal purposes have direct benefits. Scientists have discovered new ways to help skin care products penetrate the basal layer, also known as the dermal/epidermal junction (DEJ). This is where the live cells are born. When a skin care product can penetrate the dermal/epidermal junction, it can target the cells before they rise to the surface, creating healthier skin.

Skin care product delivery systems are offered by either over-the-counter (OTC) product lines or professional grade products. Most products purchased OTC sit on the skin's surface and cannot penetrate the barrier of the stratum corneum. However, professional grade product lines are developed by cosmetic chemists and contain a higher amount of active ingredients to reach deeper skin levels. These higher-level ingredients used in professional grade products are developed by cosmetic chemists. Therefore, these products can only be applied by specially trained and licensed estheticians. When highly active ingredients are encapsulated, the product can penetrate through the epidermal junction, release the ingredients from the capsule and then target the live cells as they are born.

When scientists develop professional skin care products, they use three mechanisms that active ingredients use to reach the live tissue: [3]

1. Active ingredients travel through the intercellular glue. (Remember, the cells are bricks and the lipids are the intercellular glue).
2. Active ingredients penetrate from cell to cell to reach deeper into the skin.
3. Active ingredients travel through openings in pathways such as sweat glands, oil glands or hair follicles.

Not all professional lines are created equal. Some use lesser quality ingredients and still call themselves professional products, yet they only remain on the skin's surface. When an active ingredient is sitting on the skin's surface, not only can it irritate the skin, but it doesn't benefit the cell renewal process. It is extremely important to exercise caution when selecting a product promising superior benefits that does not contain toxic or harmful ingredients. Finding the right OTC, professional or physician strength product for you will help keep your skin healthy and beautiful.

VARIOUS DELIVERY SYSTEMS

Here are some delivery systems that have been used over the years:

Dermabrasion

Frequency: Occasional

Purpose: Remove scarring, treat acne and remove deep wrinkles.

Process: A wire brush or diamond wheel removes the entire epidermis.

Benefits: Reduces deep acne scars and minimizes deep wrinkles.

Caution: The skin is raw, peeling and oozing. During the healing process, petroleum jelly is applied to keep the skin moist while it rebuilds itself. Staying indoors is a requirement to prevent skin damage, which would cause permanent, uneven colored skin.

The Skinny from Samantha

Dermabrasion literally removes the entire epidermis, leaving the skin raw and in need of major "downtime." Downtime means you need to avoid the sun for at least six weeks. Even walking to your car from the grocery store can cause the skin to burn. This would result in uneven skin tone. In addition, everyone who has had this service always has a line of demarcation on the neck where the dermabrasion treatment ended.

Laser Treatments

Frequency: 4-6 weeks

Purpose: Open holes in the skin for the product to penetrate the dermis.

Process: Laser treatment of the entire face.

Benefits: Decreases uneven skin tone, diminishes fine lines, reduces acne scarring.

Caution: Laser treatments create a thermal ablation, which heats the skin to create holes for the product to penetrate to the dermis. Depending on the laser and the depth of its light, the healing process can be the same as dermabrasion. However, newer lasers no longer remove the skin's surface or create damage as it heals. This service can be done on a lunch break.

The Skinny from Samantha

Lasers have great benefits for certain skin conditions. For deep acne scarring and deep wrinkles, these treatments are great. The problem is that the skin needs the right products to support the healing process. If not, desired results will not occur.

Microneedling

Frequency: 8 weeks

Purpose: To stimulate collagen renewal and enhance product penetration.

Process: NOTE - Microneedling is NOT allowed in some states! Needles are used to puncture the skin, which creates a controlled skin injury.

Benefits: Reduces acne scarring, fine lines and wrinkles.

The Skinny from Samantha

Microneedling has great benefits, but it also creates wounds to the skin. Microneedling works well in pushing products deeper into the skin, but newer technologies do not require such harsh trauma to the skin's surface and can achieve the same or better results.

Iontophoresis

Frequency: 4 weeks

Purpose: Ions enhance product penetration.

Process: Uses electrical current to drive charged molecules across the skin.

Benefits: Heals acne or inflamed skin.

Caution: I learned this technique in esthetics school, but it is not commonly used.

The Skinny from Samantha

Iontophoresis is taught in esthetics school to prepare the skin for acne extraction and inflammation reduction. I have only used this service while in school.

Electroporation

Frequency: 4 weeks

Purpose: Pulse of electricity briefly opens the pores to allow product to penetrate the cell membrane.

Process: Short, high-voltage electrical pulses create disruptions in the skin to allow products to penetrate.

Benefits: Reduces signs of aging, evens skin tone and increases hydration to the cells.

Caution: Do not use if you have any metal implants or pacemakers, are pregnant, or have the following conditions: active acne, heavily exfoliated skin, skin cancer, tattoos, vascular injuries or skin irritations such as eczema or dermatitis.

The Skinny from Samantha

I am familiar with this treatment, but have not had experience using it on my clients.

Ultrasound

Frequency: 4 weeks

Purpose: Enhances product penetration, gently exfoliates the skin and removes superficial blackheads (especially on the nose).

Process: High or low frequency devices, which are safe to use.

Benefits: I do an ultrasonic facial in my spa when a client has thick skin or a lot of dead skin build-up. It really helps reduce the discomfort level during extractions. A soft, gentle vibration disrupts the skin to allow product penetration.

Caution: Pacemakers are contraindicated.

The Skinny from Samantha

I love ultrasound treatments during the facial. For clients with a lot of oil in their pores, it removes the oil to make extractions easier and less painful for the client. It can also gently enhance product penetration. I have used ultrasound in both the medi-spa and my own spa. It is very relaxing and offers a gentle vibration on the skin to exfoliate and penetrate.

Chapter 3:

Proper Methods and Products for Cleansing, Treating and Moisturizing

The skin is the only organ that sees daylight. In addition to constant exposure to dirt, environmental pollutants and toxic ingredients, it is stripped, pulled, tightened and caked with makeup daily. If you think about all that the skin goes through from day to day, it is easy to recognize it as a remarkable organ. Taking care of our skin is very important. The number one client rule in my spa is the 12/353 rule. Throughout the course of a year, 365 days, I see my clients 12 times a year for facials, and I do not see my clients for the remaining 353 days of the year. That means how they care for their skin on those 353 days is what makes the biggest impact on their appearance.

 What are you doing on 353 days of the year? Washing two times per day! Right?

Are you someone who falls asleep on the couch, gets tired at night, or you just don't feel like doing one more thing? After a long day, it's easy to forget to wash the face and climb right into bed to catch some z's. However, washing your face before going to bed is the single most important action you can take each day to ensure your skin stays healthy and youthful looking. While you sleep, your skin repairs itself, so it must be properly cleansed to reap the full benefit of the repair mode.

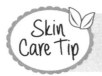 Skin should never feel tight and squeaky-clean. If it does, it is a sign that your cleanser is too harsh.

A few years ago, my sister shared a Facebook post about a woman who deliberately slept in her makeup for 30 days to see the impact on her skin. *In 30 days, her skin dulled, broke out with acne, caused uneven skin tone, highlighted dark patches and deepened wrinkles.*[4] Regardless of how tired you are at night, wash your face before settling down for the evening to capitalize on every minute of repair.

PROPER FACE WASHING

Face washing is the most important step in your daily skin care routine. Massaging the cleanser all over the face stimulates circulation, allowing the product to penetrate deeper into the skin, thereby increasing its effectiveness in reaching the dermal/epidermal junction.

True or False Washing Tips

1. Don't wash your face after a workout.
2. If you wash in the morning, you do not have to wash at night.
3. If you wash at night, just splash water on your face in the morning.
4. Use any soap product you have within reach.
5. Exfoliate every day.

If you answered false to all of the above, you win! Read the following tips for the accurate answers.

TRUE & FALSE EXPLANATIONS - EFFECTIVE TIPS TO CLEANSE THE FACE

Response to Question #1 - Always wash after every workout.
Exercise is very important to stay healthy, strong and keep all the organs working properly. During a workout, two million sweat glands act as the body's personal air conditioning system. Sweat is mostly water, but also contains a mixture of minerals such as sodium, potassium, calcium, magnesium and urea. *Interestingly, none of the contents of sweat stink; it's the bacteria on your skin's surface that interacts with sweat produced by the apocrine glands to produce the smell.*[5]

I used to drag my kids to the gym for morning workouts. Since I was already out, I ran errands and returned home in time for lunch and naps. Most of the time, I found myself still needing a shower around dinnertime.

It is extremely important to wash the face within 20 minutes of exercising to remove the sweat off the skin. Those who do not wash after a workout tend to have a lot of little bumps or small red pimples on the forehead caused by clogged pores that mixed with dirt and oil. When sweat sits on the skin hours after a workout, it can cause various skin conditions to develop including acne, rosacea and dry skin. Be sure to wash and apply sunscreen after each wash and before any workout or activity that makes you sweat such as gardening, biking, etc.

For those hectic days, keep baby wipes in your car for moments you can't fully wash and shower. Baby wipes are gentler than facial cleansing cloths. Occasional use of these cloths will do in a pinch to at least remove the sweat. Do not use on a regular basis and not daily. Many facial cleansing cloths have irritating or toxic ingredients that strip the skin of oil, irritate the skin and don't clean it properly.

Responses to Questions #2 & #3 - Wash Your Face Every Night and Every Morning
Studies show that in order to maintain a healthy lifestyle, the body

needs eight hours of sleep to repair and renew itself. After 10pm, the body repairs itself; any later, and the repair time is decreased. Like sleep benefits, washing the face before bed is just as important as the required number of hours for sleep. The skin cannot properly repair itself when it is caked with makeup, dirt, oil and sweat. When you forget to wash at night, it accelerates the aging process, damages the skin and creates clogged pores, which lead to breakouts.

Skin Care Tip

1. Wash with cleanser in the morning and the evening. A splash of water does not clean well enough.
2. Use clean cloths so that the dirt from the previous use does not return to the face. A microfiber cloth is very gentle on the skin.
3. Be sure to wash the entire face, especially along the hairline. Hair products clog the skin and can result in little white bumps.
4. Rinse thoroughly. Residual cleanser can lead to build-up and develop bumps or blackheads.

Responses to Questions #4 & #5 -
The Proper Facial Cleanser and Exfoliator

There is a plethora of cleansers on the market. Gel, foamy or creamy cleansers work to treat different skin types. Some even have scrubs within the cleanser. The wrong cleanser strips the skin of natural oils, dehydrates it or creates sensitivities.

- Gel cleansers are good for acne or oily skin types.
- Foamy cleansers are great for oily to normal skin types or drier skins in the summer when the weather is humid.
- Creamy cleansers work for dry skin and even normal to oily during the dry, winter months.
- There is no need for the cleanser to include scrubs or exfoliants!
- Most over-the-counter (OTC) facial cleansers contain irritating ingredients or exfoliation scrubs or glycolic acids.

SABRINA'S STORY

Let's face it. Whether a mom, career woman, or both, we are busy. No matter the type of work we do, stress, lack of sleep, eating on the go, caffeine intake and hormones do not treat our bodies kindly on the inside, nor the outside. Does this sound like you? It happens to all of us. Meet seriously busy Sabrina.

After a crazy week, the mirror reflects all the points of the big dipper on her pretty face. Wearing a cape, Sabrina dashes to the store to buy an acne cleanser and save the day. She grabs the bottle that stands out the most and screams 'helps control breakouts.' A sigh of relief escapes as she quickly glances at the front label and notices 'bonus scrub' or 'glycolic acid' or 'salicylic acid.' "That should do the trick."

Immediately, she zooms back home, washes and commits to the right regimen - cleansing both morning and night. A few days later, the little dipper appears next to the big dipper, her face is sensitive and now even dryer. After six weeks or so of this constant battle, Sabrina gives up and finds her local, trusted and licensed esthetician referred by many friends. She makes the call that will change everything. For her appointment, she brings all the products she is currently using.

What happened? Here's the Scoop.

Applying a product to your skin with known skin irritants or with exfoliation ingredients is too much for your skin. The skin disagrees with that product and the skin becomes:

- stripped and compromised
- dry because it is no longer able to retain moisture
- filled with microtears which allow bacteria, dirt, environmental toxins and UV rays to enter our skin
- unable to penetrate the skin's barrier and enter the bloodstream, which also supplies our skin cells in the dermis
- a pathway to compromise the internal body system
- excessively dry and rapidly losing moisture because the skin can't keep up

This is a vicious cycle and the skin knows that if it continues to function like this, both the dead skin cells that offer protection and the water that offers moisture will dissipate. The bloodstream must work extra hard to eliminate the harmful ingredients so they don't damage the other organs in our body. However, I am in awe of the skin because its most remarkable aspect is that it protects itself from all this damage.

The skin creates inflammation and "plumps" itself up to give itself an added layer of protection while it fixes the damage caused by the wrong product. If we pay attention, the skin will tell us if something is not working. The condition may worsen. When the skin is swollen, we notice that our pore size is smaller, our wrinkles aren't as deep and the skin looks more "plump and youthful." That is not the case! The skin is actually fighting to keep itself intact by creating its own inflammation.

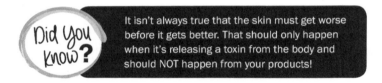

Did you know? It isn't always true that the skin must get worse before it gets better. That should only happen when it's releasing a toxin from the body and should NOT happen from your products!

When our skin is inflamed, it is damaged. The only way to fix this damage is to stop using harsh, irritating, and toxic products. Find a professional skin care line from a trusted esthetician who will customize your products to fit your skin's needs. It may take some time in the beginning, especially if you've been compromising your skin's barrier for many years. The skin has a memory and will eventually restore itself, but damage done over many years will result in older-looking skin. Don't worry, your esthetician will guide you and keep track of your skin and home care products so you can repair the damage and help your skin as you age.

Lessons Learned from Sabrina

First, daily exfoliation is too much stimulation. Exfoliants can be in the form of scrubs, alpha-hydroxy acids (AHA's) such as glycolic acid or lactic acid, retinols and mechanical scrubbing brushes. Many of these products are added to facial cleansers and recommended for use both morning and night. For women with dry, acne prone skin like Sabrina, these ingredients strip the skin and create excessive dryness. Then, her skin becomes desensitized from the irritating ingredients she is putting on her face morning and night.

No need to exfoliate every day. The skin is a natural exfoliator.

We shouldn't be over-exfoliating. Our skin naturally sheds itself every 28 days, and as we age, it can take 45-60 or more days. The natural exfoliation process protects the skin by exfoliating only when new cells are ready. Forcing this process requires the skin to work harder to protect itself. When the skin is over-exfoliated, the skin protects itself by swelling, which in turn, causes inflammation. Too much exfoliation can also increase sensitivity. This is where the importance of an esthetician comes in.

When Sabrina comes to my spa, I analyze her skin by looking at and touching her skin to feel the level of dryness. The dryness could be due to using an acne cleanser that is made for oily skin. Depending upon the season, I use a foamy or creamy cleanser. We talk diet, fluctuating hormones and lifestyle for which I offer her alternatives to healthy, easy on-the-go snacks and tips to de-stress. I see her monthly to check her progress and adjust her at-home skin care products to keep her skin healthy, hydrated and free from breakouts.

It is amazing how quickly the skin responds and repairs itself after switching from an irritating cleanser to one that works best for a specific skin type. A licensed and trusted esthetician can give advice and check ingredients in the products used at home.

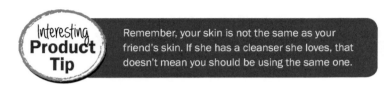

Interesting Product Tip

Remember, your skin is not the same as your friend's skin. If she has a cleanser she loves, that doesn't mean you should be using the same one.

EXFOLIATING WITH ENZYMES

Enzymes are the second most important product to have in your beauty routine. I have observed significant improved results on my clients' skin and my own. SPF is the first. In this chapter, I will talk about the benefit of enzymes and how to use them properly.

Enzymes are made up of either papain (papaya), bromelain (pineapple) or berries which are fruit-based products. When eaten, these fruits have great health benefits. They are also great for our skin because our skin needs the nutrients to stay hydrated and to increase hydration in the cells.

Enzymes are beneficial to our skin because their main job is to eat proteins. Our skin cells are made of protein. As they rise to the skin's surface and die, they lose their cell components and the protein from the cell is left behind. Enzymes eat these proteins (dead skin cells that are no longer needed) to give the skin a light, gentle exfoliation that keeps the skin cells shedding properly as we age. Once the enzymes have done their job, hydrated the skin with nutrients from the fruit enzymes, your moisturizer can now get to the skin and do its job.

Most spas sell enzymes in their professional line of products. Ask your esthetician for recommendations. Be careful of over-the-counter (OTC) enzymes because some of them do have scrubs, AHAs or harsh ingredients that can strip the skin. Check ingredient labels, and when in doubt, seek out the advice of a trusted esthetician.

It's not hard or even time consuming to use enzymes, and your reflection will reward you for the time spent on it. All it requires is:

- Wash your face and rinse off the cleanser.
- Apply a pea-sized amount of the enzyme to your hands.
- Massage it into your face. Massage stimulates your circulation but also stimulates the enzyme to start working and dissolve the proteins on your skin.
- Let it sit for 5-10 minutes while you shower and rinse off the enzyme at the end.
- Apply your serum, if applicable.
- Apply your SPF moisturizer.
- Your skin looks and feels great the entire day.

Samantha's Cleanse

With my clients, I make sure that every single client no longer uses AHAs, BHAs, scrubs or mechanical scrubbing brushes that are harsh, strip the skin of moisture or cause dehydration. The enzymes naturally replace the need for any of these products.

We are all tired by the end of the day. The last thing we want to do at night is run back and forth to the bathroom washing, applying the enzyme, and running back to rinse it off and moisturize. I feel the same way, which is why I keep mine in the shower. I suggest my clients do the same and apply the enzyme just once a week for 5-10 minutes. The results are so worth it.

SERUMS – SKIN CARE'S GREATEST SECRET

Serums are created to treat the skin and repair specific skin conditions, such as acne, rosacea and melasma. Vitamin A, in its natural form, is called retinaldehyde and is non-irritating. When penetrated properly, it is one of the best treatment serums on the market. Serums are dependent upon the skin and the willingness of my clients to use them. I have many clients who use serums daily. Others don't want to add in extra steps because they prefer a simple routine. Serums are important, but if you're not willing to commit, buying a serum is a waste of money. Most likely, you will never use it or else you will use it so infrequently, it will spoil. You may end up putting expired product on your skin, which will cause more harm.

A serum is designed for penetration to occur. Active ingredients are unstable unless encapsulated. Cosmetic chemists have found a way to encapsulate them (put them in a bubble) to hold their active state and stabilize them. Serums therefore can be massaged into the skin to penetrate to the dermal/epidermal junction (DEJ) where the live cells are born. When the product reaches the DEJ, the active ingredients can nourish your skin and repair DNA damage.

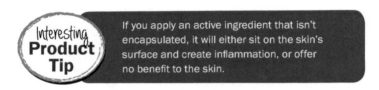

Interesting **Product Tip**

If you apply an active ingredient that isn't encapsulated, it will either sit on the skin's surface and create inflammation, or offer no benefit to the skin.

Not all serums are created equal! There is an ongoing theme here for you to notice. OTC serums are not the same as professional serums because there are fewer active ingredients and more fillers and preservatives. OTC serums also lack the delivery system to the DEJ which causes them to remain on top of the skin. This does not help to improve the skin's condition, and it may even create inflammation.

OTC serums can cause inflammation. Inflammation puffs out the skin which makes it appear clearer and healthy. However, underneath, it is suffering and is working hard to repair itself. When people don't know this, the before and after pictures used in advertising look attractive, as if the serum does cure the skin. Unfortunately, the skin is in the inflammation stage.

Professional serums are made in smaller batches and contain fewer fillers because estheticians want to see your skin conditions improve. Scientists behind professional skin care lines are either estheticians who have become cosmetic chemists or they are physicians who design products for estheticians. These products are results-based and use ingredients in a way that the skin will accept and absorb the ingredients into the skin.

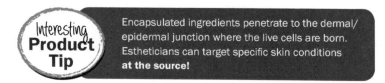

Interesting Product Tip

Encapsulated ingredients penetrate to the dermal/epidermal junction where the live cells are born. Estheticians can target specific skin conditions **at the source!**

Estheticians can now use serums with a carrier that encapsulates the active ingredients into a "bubble." The encapsulated ingredient can penetrate to the DEJ for release where the live cells are born. This means that we can target specific skin conditions at their source to effectively treat the skin.

As a serum, Vitamin C is a great example of different dosages for skin care. On the ingredient label, it is usually listed as ascorbic acid, ascorbyl phosphate, ascorbyl palmitate or L-ascorbic acid. The front of the label may say 'Antioxidant Serum' or 'Vitamin C to reduce dark spots.' Be aware, if L-ascorbic acid is not listed as one of the first five ingredients, it is not true Vitamin C.

When reading a product label, ingredients are listed in order from the most to least amounts. Manufacturers will trick consumers by stating there is an active ingredient in a serum, but when you look at the ingredient list, the serum is at the bottom of the label. (See how to read labels in Chapter 7.)

Read labels, and if you are unsure, ask your esthetician for help to target concerns. A good esthetician will keep track of your skin and adjust your serums based on how your skin is progressing. Customized serums can help you reach your skin care goals.

MASKS

For decades, masks have been part of the skin care regimen. With good skin care habits and products, masks are no longer an essential item. When seeing an esthetician regularly, which is about once a month, each treatment ends with a mask. One mask per month is enough. However, some people still like the routine and benefits a mask offers. For you, I share the following information.

At-Home Facial Masks

Masks used at home are in one of three categories: pore-clearing or clay-based; creamy; or gel. Each mask is best for one specific type of skin condition. The caveat is when using it for one condition, additional conditions may not be addressed and those conditions could worsen.

Pore-Clearing or Clay-Based Masks

These masks are designed for acne, for oily skin or for large pores filled with blackheads. Most of these masks are sulfur-based because of the ingredient's anti-bacterial and anti-microbial properties. Sulfur helps decrease the effect of acne bacteria on the skin, is very calming and reduces acne inflammation during active breakouts. Clay masks are drying and should not be used on dry or sensitive skins. *Note: Clay masks that contains kaolin gently remove the surface oil and dirt from pores. It will not remove the blackhead itself, but it will prevent a blackhead from forming. Kaolin is also a calming ingredient that cleanses and decreases the size of pores.*

Creamy masks

These masks are beneficial for dry, dehydrated and sometimes, even acne or rosacea. Cream-based masks are more hydrating and offer the skin a layer of moisture when removed. Cream masks do not feel tight as they dry and are easy to remove. *Note: If you have T-zone oil (combination skin), these types of masks will not address pores or control the blackheads. Some cream masks may actually cause blackheads because they can be occlusive, which means as they dry, moisture is sealed into the skin, or they contain ingredients that cause blackheads.*

Gel masks

Gel masks calm and soothe the skin while offering an anti-inflammatory action. They are best for those with rosacea or sensitive skin because the gel is cooling and calms the redness. Be sure to check ingredients because some gel masks can irritate the skin, especially acne gel masks. *Note: Those using prescription acne products or OTC acne lines may suffer from dehydrated skin.*

Using a mask at home is a personal preference. If you regularly receive treatments from an esthetician, it may be redundant. Discuss at-home masks with her to see if a customized mask can be created to meet your at-home needs.

MOISTURIZING YOUR SKIN

Moisturizing is an important step to keeping your skin feeling moist and preventing water loss from the skin. Moisturizers act as a sealant on your skin to seal in moisture and prevent moisture from evaporating. I always suggest a night time moisturizer in the evening and a sunscreen moisturizer in the morning. You need SPF EVERY day. When necessary, I may add a facial oil or boosting oil-based moisturizer on top of the moisturizer to give the skin that added layer of protection and hydrate the oil glands. It can either be added on top of the moisturizer or mixed together with the moisturizer. Some of the common ingredient categories for moisturizers include emulsions, humectants, emollients, preservatives and surfactants.

Lotions & Creams

When lotions and creams are applied to the skin, the water typically evaporates and leaves the remainder of the mixture to do its job. Creams are heavier than lotions and sometimes, when the emulsifier is mixed, it becomes oil-in-water, which means that the consistency is heavier and will leave a film on the skin. This is great for dry skin because the product remains water-resistant and maintains the hydration level of the skin.

Lotions tend to use water-in-oil formulations because these products are designed for oily, combination and normal skin types. When the skin is oily, you do need oil to maintain the balance of oil production, but not to the extent of a moisturizing cream. Water-in-oil formulations tend to be lighter in consistency than creams which can feel thick and heavy.

Moisturizers are formulated one of two ways: water-in-oil or oil-in-water. Considering that oil and water don't mix, it seems peculiar that these ingredients compose the formulas. To prevent separation, emulsifiers are added to maintain the equality of the water-in-oil and to stabilize the two ingredients which prevent separation. An easy way to understand this process is to examine a common emulsifier, mayonnaise. Basic mayonnaise is made with vegetable oil, eggs and water. *The lecithin from the egg keeps the oil and water together in a nice, white, thick emulsion.*[6]

Occlusive Moisturizers

Occlusive moisturizers are thicker in nature to create a barrier on the skin's surface and seal moisture into the skin. Dimethicone and petroleum or mineral oil (derived from petroleum) are occlusive ingredients. Petroleum is controversial because it is a by-product and mineral oil is known to clog the skin. Dimethicone has received a bad rap as well. However, dimethicone is a large molecule and cannot penetrate the skin's barrier, which means it sits on the skin's surface. For clients that suffer from dry or dehydrated skin, this is good because it seals moisture into the skin, almost like applying saran wrap.

Those with acne, oily skin or who tend to breakout easily should not use occlusive moisturizers.

Ingredients for Moisturizers

Next to applying the moisturizer, the next important step is finding the right product. There are pros and cons to the ingredients in moisturizers. When reading a product label, the first ingredient in a moisturizer should always be water; this is typical in water-in-oil moisturizers. The moisture part is called a "humectant" which attracts moisture to the skin and retains it in the stratum corneum, the top layer of the epidermis.

Emulsifiers

Emulsifiers prevent a product from separating because they act as a binder to keep the oil-in-water products from separating in the product. Think about creating a salad dressing of oil and vinegar. The dressing needs to be stirred or shaken to combine the ingredients, but after a few minutes, they begin to separate again. In skin care products, there are oil-soluble and water-soluble ingredients and both add benefits to the skin to keep it hydrated. Moisturizers need both oil-soluble and water-soluble ingredients because the oil keeps the oil glands hydrated.

Emulsifiers have skin-clogging potential, so avoid or practice minimize usage with them if you have oily skin or are acne-prone. When reading labels, emulsifiers are listed as an ingredient with a hyphen followed by a number. Common emulsifier ingredients considered safe include Steareth-21 or Ceteareth-20. Cosmetic chemists also need to track the amount of emulsifier used. Too much of this ingredient will sit on the skin's surface and cause irritation.

Emollients

Emollients are used to make moisturizers spreadable on the skin. They help soften and smooth the skin, and they also form a protective layer on the skin's surface to prevent moisture loss. Some common emollient ingredients include lanolin and cetyl alcohol.

Preservatives

Preservatives are very important in any product because they protect products from growing bacteria, mold, and fungus, which can be more harmful to our skin and bodies than certain ingredients. Over-the-counter (OTC) products use more preservatives than professional grade products because OTC products are made in large batches and are formulated to sit on a warehouse shelf for up to two years before it hits the store. Since professional products are made in smaller batches, the formula requires fewer preservatives. Professional products must be used within six months of opening or the preservatives and active ingredients within the product can expire. If a product expires, never use it because it can damage the skin or create sensitivities.

Parabens

Parabens used to be the most commonly used preservative in products and some lines still use them. Much controversy surrounds the use of parabens and research continues. *Dr. Philip W. Harvey Ph.D., registered toxicologist at Covance Laboratories, Ltd. in the United Kingdom says, "The whole area is poorly researched, but now it's time to coordinate funding and support in a few key areas of environmental endocrine disruption and human health, and the cosmetics scenario is one of the most promising to study in a controlled way. It is easy to say that there is no evidence of parabens or cosmetics being associated with a health effect if the research has not been done; indeed, the statement is misleading to the public."[7]*

Dr. Ben Johnson, president, founder and formulator of Osmosis Skin Care explains, "any ingredients, such as parabens, that have the ability to form a tumor should never be used." Johnson does not support parabens and does not use them in his products. However, there are many chemists who use parabens and feel that they are the most effective preservative. *(See Chapter 7 for more information on parabens.)*

Some other commonly used preservatives are phenoxyethanol, methylisothiazolinone, DMDM hydanatoin and diazolidinyl urea. Many of these ingredients are not very good ingredients and are explained in more detail in Chapter 7. The ones that are considered good to use include benzyl alcohol, citric acid, and xanthan gum.

Surfactants

Lastly, surfactants are used to lift away oil and dirt from the skin. Their role is also to improve the spread ability of a product. *Some common surfactant ingredients include polyethylene glycols (PEG's). These are condensed polymers of ethylene oxide used for a wide range of purposes in cosmetics depending on molecular weight.*[8]

When searching for a moisturizer, be mindful of ingredients by reading labels, but also check with your esthetician. Make sure that your moisturizer doesn't have comedogenic ingredients hidden in the label, which will clog your pores and either cause or worsen acne. Depending on the season and your skin type, estheticians know how to customize moisturizers to keep your skin hydrated no matter the season.

DAYTIME AND NIGHT TIME SKIN CARE ROUTINES

You now know how important it is to wash your face both morning and night. The most effective practice to healthy skin is a consistent routine. The following recommended regimen is a basic skin care schedule which will help you look and feel good even when you don't have skin conditions to manage. With or without conditions, many still worry about aging or maintaining their current youthful look. Consistent skin care practices can help with these issues.

Morning Routine

The goals for the morning routine are to cleanse and protect. Using products with active ingredients will target specific skin conditions, like acne, rosacea and melasma. Your esthetician will be able to help fine-tune your morning routine based on your specific skin's needs.

1. Wash your face with a cleanser.
2. Apply a recommended serum that is higher in vitamin C or can help hydrate the skin. Depending on the severity of your skin condition, you may or may not want to use your active serums in the morning.
3. Use a chemical-free, zinc oxide-based SPF moisturizer.

4. Exfoliate only 1-2 times a week, depending on the weather and your skin type.

Night Time Routine

At night time, cleansing prepares the skin to repair itself during sleep. Plan accordingly, and don't skip because you are too tired. This is a crucial step in your skin care routine.

1. Wash your face with a cleanser. The same cleanser can be used both morning and night.
2. Avoid daily scrubs.
3. Apply enzymes up to twice a week depending on esthetician's recommendations.
4. It is crucial to apply a serum at night. A professional level active serum gives it an added boost of treatment to heal new cells forming at the dermal/epidermal junction (DEJ). Peptides, stem cell serums, exosomes and vitamin A are four effective ingredients that should be applied to the skin in the form of a serum at night. *Note: Depending on the source, these ingredients can either make a dramatic difference or do nothing.*
5. Massage the entire face and neck with a good night moisturizer. This moisturizer should be a little heavier than your daytime one and no SPF is needed. Night moisturizers have more hydrating ingredients that sit on the skin's surface and prevent moisture-loss. Ideally, the job of a moisturizer is to sit on the skin's surface. The serums penetrate the surface, and the moisturizer keeps the skin soft, supple and moist. A proper night moisturizer will act like a blanket that prevents water from evaporating off the skin.

It takes time to get used to a morning and night time routine. After a short while, it will become second nature and give you noticeable results. If you need help or have any questions, seek advice from your esthetician. Our job is to keep your skin healthy and customize your at-home skin care routine to fit your needs and your schedule.

SPECIAL CARE FOR EYES, LIPS, NECK

So far, we have covered morning and night time routines, how to best cleanse and moisturize. The next step is to learn about the three areas that need extra special TLC: the eyes, lips and neck. The structure for the eyes, lips and neck are different than the skin on the rest of the body. Due to their delicate nature, they need extra special care when selecting ingredients and applying products.

Eye Care

The eyes are the windows to the soul. The eye area is very sensitive and the skin is much thinner than the rest of the face. Different from other areas of the body, the eye area does not have oil glands that protect the skin to keep it lubricated. Therefore, as we mature, eyes are the first things we notice changing. Whether it is dark, puffy circles, thin, crepe paper-like texture or the first wrinkles (also known as crow's feet), these changes can be improved.

Puffy Eyes

The skin surrounding the eyes is very sensitive, extremely thin and filled with blood vessels. Under eye puffiness can be caused by two common factors:

1. Fluid retention, the most common cause, which can be minimized by limiting salt, managing seasonal allergies, and sinus congestion. Using an eye cream will increase circulation and decrease inflammation.
2. Herniated fat is less common and can only be treated by surgery.

Puffiness or Dark Circles

These two conditions are usually related, especially if it's not a direct result from the capillaries. Causes can stem from:

- Lack of sleep
- Allergies, colds and sinus issues which increase fluid to the face and can get stuck under the eyes (which is why allergies can present themselves as swollen eyes)
- Using the wrong products; some OTC eye creams won't help decrease fluid or dark circles

- Makeup and removing makeup
- Excessive caffeine or alcohol consumption
- Imbalance in our body

Lack of Sleep

Sleeping less than eight hours will result in dark circles under the eyes. Most of us have experienced the dark circles at one time or another.

Vasodilators

Caffeine and alcohol cause puffy eyes because as vasodilators, they constrict the blood vessels. Once the alcohol or caffeine leaves our system, our blood vessels plump up and fill with oxygen to compensate for the decrease. Surprisingly, it only takes one glass of wine or a bottle of beer to constrict our blood vessels, especially if we consume either within an hour of going to bed. As for caffeine, it includes coffee, soft drinks, energy drinks, chocolate and even some undereye creams, which contain coffee.

Samantha's Cleanse

Have you ever stopped using an OTC anti-aging product and noticed the wrinkles come back or your skin looks older? That is the result of skin damage from using improper products that create surface inflammation. This process causes the skin to age more quickly than normal, which is why consumers then see a dermatologist or visit a medi-spa for injectables. Using some of these products can damage the skin. Depending on how long you have used them, the damage may not be reparable or reversible.

Ok, I'm off my soap box! I will now discuss the benefits of why you should choose professional skin care products from your favorite esthetician!

Wrong Products

Many of the OTC eye products use inflammatory ingredients that can contribute to dry, thin skin. If you are already sensitive, you are only making the eye area worse. Ingredients like alpha-hydroxy acids (AHA's), retinols, propylene glycol or even the fragrances and preservatives can irritate and inflame the eye area.

Peptides, hyaluronic acid, seaweed and chlorella vulgaris (if you're not allergic to iodine) are good to use for under the eyes for anti-aging and to decrease inflammation.

Imbalance of Toxins in the Body
Solving an imbalance is a relatively easy thing to do first thing in the morning with a lukewarm glass of water and a slice of lemon. Lemon acts as a neutralizer for the body and gets our digestive system moving. Lemon water also acts as an anti-inflammatory agent, so it decreases puffiness in the body and the eye area.

Dark Circles, Wrinkles & Aging
The eye area tends to be dry, and therefore, more prone to dark circles and wrinkling. Darkness is caused from capillaries or blood vessels, which show up as purple under the eyes. An eye treatment in the spa soothes and reduces wrinkles, puffiness, dark circles or thin skin. Gently exfoliating the dead skin cells decreases inflammation and lightens the darkness under the eyes.

APPLYING EYE CREAM & MAKEUP

Makeup
Another reason our eye area ages faster is how we remove our makeup. Think about how you do it. Do you use a facial cleansing cloth (with irritating ingredients) or do you rub your eyes to get rid of every last drop of mascara to avoid looking like a raccoon? Either way, most of us use friction to remove makeup. Pulling the delicate skin leads to more wrinkles. The friction irritates the eye area, and breaks delicate capillaries.

Removing Makeup

- Find a professional level makeup remover that is gentle to the skin. Be cautious of OTC products using irritating ingredients, such as sodium lauryl sulfate, propylene glycol, mineral oil and fragrance. My spa carries a gel-based remover that you gently massage into the eyes and rinse off - no pulling or scrubbing needed.
- Jojoba oil will not clog your pores because there are no oil glands.
- Be sure to keep the area hydrated with a professional eye cream, both morning and night, after removing your makeup.
- When applying your eye products or removing your makeup, you ALWAYS want to go with the grain (i.e. remove the makeup towards your nose). This avoids pulling on the delicate skin, which creates deeper wrinkles.

Eye Cream

The ring finger is the best finger to apply eye products because it is the weakest and will not put too much pressure on the area. Dab a pin-sized amount of product on one ring finger; then dab both ring fingers together to share the product. Start on the temple and gently pat the product onto the brow bone – NOT directly under the eye. The reason is because when we blink our eyes, our product can move and if it's too close, it can get into your eyes and irritate them. By putting your product on the brow bone, blinking will move it into the under-eye area and not into the actual eye.

Makeup

To hide dark circles, apply a concealer onto the inner eye area. Again, dab a pin-sized amount onto your ring finger. Tap on the spot where your eyebrow begins and follow along the inner eye area along the nose to mid-eye area underneath. Repeat until all concealer has been tapped into the skin.

Lip Care

The lips have the same skin layers as the rest of the skin on our bodies. However, the lips are highly sensitive because they have no oil, no sweat glands, nor hair follicles to give us protection from the elements. Our lips are also constantly exposed to our saliva, which dries them out. Once our lips are dry, it is very hard to rehydrate them. Keeping our lips wet is not the solution; it only makes the dryness worse!

We usually apply chap stick to combat dry lips, but have you ever noticed that no matter how much you use, your lips always feel dry? The ingredients in chap sticks can be irritating. In addition, some contain parabens, or unnecessary preservatives, that are not healthy for lips, skin or body. Unfortunately, these ingredients are ingested as we eat while wearing the product.

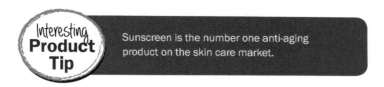

Interesting **Product Tip**

Sunscreen is the number one anti-aging product on the skin care market.

Lips are just as susceptible to sun damage as the rest of our faces, and although, not common, applying SPF is a must. Fortunately, lip balms and chap stick have started to include SPF in their products. It's always good to check ingredients to prevent using products that irritate, dry or contain chemical sunscreen ingredients.

Neck Care

The neck is one of the most neglected areas of our skin and therefore more susceptible to folding, sagging, deepened lines and wrinkles. The lines can run either horizontally or vertically depending on the damage to the skin. Age, genetics, skin composition and lifestyle impact how your neck will age. If your mom or grandma had thin skin on their necks, you may also be prone to the same issues as you age. Unfortunately, when the neck isn't treated the same as the face, a woman's age is noticeable.

Tips for Neck Care
1. Cleanse thoroughly during the morning or night routines.

2. Apply serums daily, as they are your worker bees. The purpose of the serum is to treat the skin as they get into the base of the epidermis where the live cells are born. Vitamin A serums (not retinols), peptides, Vitamin C and hyaluronic acid are all serum ingredients which should be used daily.

3. Moisturize. If your skin tends to be dry, add some of your night moisturizer to your daily SPF to give your neck some added moisture. Reapply moisturizer throughout the day if you still feel dry. This area needs extra moisture and TLC, so don't skip the neck!

4. Don't forget the SPF. Sunscreen is the number one anti-aging product on the skin care market. Skin composition is improved by using quality products and continuously applying sunscreen.

Part 2: Healthy Inside Out

Chapter 4:

Internal Factors Influencing Skin Conditions

We discussed in Part 1 that the skin is an organ of the body. Did you know that the skin is the only organ that we can touch? This means that our skin is connected to all our internal organs and is literally like a map. Many estheticians are now learning about Face Mapping to help identify which organ in the body is imbalanced. Like Chinese medicine, where the hands and feet map the body, our face can indicate certain skin conditions on the face or back.

We are finally able to properly treat skin suffering from acne, rosacea and melasma. We can help our clients clear up their skin for good, if they are compliant and follow every recommendation we offer. Once the skin is clear, there is no need to wear heavy concealer and foundation to hide those imperfections whenever we leave the house.

The result is less time spent in front of the mirror, which makes for happier clients and estheticians! If you are happy and loving your skin, we are happy because we helped you get there without using medication nor harsh skin care products, but just loving, results-based facials!

Our face is the most exposed part of our body and encounters the most wear and tear. The skin on the face is thinner than the rest of our bodies. This is also why the face shows pimples, redness and uneven skin tone. The back is next to show skin problems because there is more friction in that area. We don't care for our backs like we do our faces or the rest of our body because we just can't reach it. The only time we think about the skin on the back is when we are suffering from acne. Have you ever wondered why only the upper back suffers from skin conditions and not the entire back? The skin is thicker from the mid-back down because we have organs, such as kidneys to protect.

Except for the décolletage, the skin on the front of our body is the thickest because it needs to protect our internal organs. For this reason, it more likely to have pimples or skin concerns from the chest down when wearing tight-fitting bras, sports bras, sweating and not washing the skin properly.

INFLAMMATION

In recent years, scientists have found a direct link between the foods in the diet and issues in the skin. Gluten, dairy and sugar are three of the worst foods consumed. These three ingredients create horrible side effects which have been found to contribute to diseases and skin problems for many people. All three of these ingredients contribute to the inflammation of our bodies.

Two Types Of Inflammation

Acute Inflammation

Acute inflammation arises after a cut or scrape in the skin, infected ingrown nail, sprained ankle, acute bronchitis, sore throat, tonsillitis or appendicitis. It is short-term and the effects subside after a few days.

Chronic Inflammation

Chronic inflammation is a long-term condition caused by habitual or environmental factors, such as excessive weight, poor diet, lack of exercise, stress, smoking, pollution, poor oral health and excessive alcohol consumption.[9]

In addition to these two types of inflammation, skin inflammation is also prevalent, and a trusted esthetician can help calm the skin to reduce the inflammation.

SKIN INFLAMMATION

The skin is an amazing organ, and its job is to protect our bodies from dirt, germs and environmental pollutants. The skin's barrier is made up of dead skin cells and has oil glands in place to produce oil and keep the skin lubricated. This oil can trap dirt from the environment into pores. The skin also knows how to protect itself from the damaging UV rays of the sun. When the skin is compromised, it is unable to properly function and protect itself, causing an inflammatory response.

Causes of Skin Inflammation

Improper Sunscreen

All sunscreens protect against UVB rays, but not always UVA rays, unless it is stated on the label. When the UV rays hit unprotected skin, the skin becomes inflamed and produces more melanin. As explained in Chapter 1, our skin darkens or tans to protect the dermis from sun damage. After repeated or lengthy sun exposure, the skin produces an inflammatory response, known as sunburn. However, the melanin cells activate and intensify. The swelling shields the cells being born at the dermal/epidermal junction.

Skin Care or Makeup Products

Oftentimes, we purchase skin care or makeup without knowing how it will interact with our skin. If the product does not match our skin's needs, it can cause inflammation and other issues. With all kinds of options like department store cosmetic counters, home party product representatives, store shelves and spas, it isn't easy to find a high-quality product that will solve your skin issues.

It's not that the product lines are all bad, but it's more about what works best for your skin. Everyone's skin is unique, and that is what makes it difficult. Even though cosmetic salespeople categorize everyone in dry, oily or combination skin types, those are not the only skin types.

Furthermore, it's hard to tell when a product is or isn't working. Frustration can sometimes set in, leading to the purchase of another product to correct the issue. A month later, after using the wrong products, the skin is worse, feels horrible, swollen and is not healing. Or sometimes it feels bad, but it looks better because the swelling has eliminated the wrinkles.

When the skin is not happy, it never quickly responds to a particular product. When this happens, your skin becomes inflamed to shield the cells in the dermis from further damage. Basically, it accelerates the aging process.

Samantha's Cleanse

Removing dead skin cells. Whenever I hear commercials or sales people say "We need to remove the dead skin cells," I cringe! This is a false statement because the skin IS dead skin cells and without it, we wouldn't have the protection our skin needs from the environment.

SYMPTOMS OF INFLAMMATION

There are several reasons the body and skin suffer from inflammation. To heal itself, the blood vessels in the body dilate so the white blood cells can target and heal the inflamed area. Inflammation has several symptoms:

- Redness
- Swelling
- Hot or warm feeling
- Pain

FOODS THAT FIGHT INFLAMMATION

There are many foods that can help fight inflammation. Abbie Major, licensed esthetician and owner of Abbie Major Skin Love says, *"Inflammation is part of the body's immune response; without it, we can't heal. But when it's out of control—as in rheumatoid arthritis—it can damage the body. Plus, it's thought to play a role in obesity, heart disease, and cancer. Foods high in sugar and saturated fat can spur inflammation and should be kept to a minimum."*[59]

Anti-inflammatory diets, such as the Paleo and Mediterranean diets, are great for bodies and skin because they work to reduce inflammation. With a focus on eating clean, your body will feel better. The best foods to eat to reduce inflammation are high amounts of fruits and vegetables, fish or grass-fed proteins. Limit red meats. Many of us go about our day and never stop to think about what our bodies are telling us. Through cravings, our body tells us if we need something nutritious or if we feel hungry. Oftentimes, the feeling of hunger is really the need to hydrate. Hunger and dehydration go hand-in-hand because many of us know that if we are thirsty, we should grab a glass of water instead of mindlessly snacking.

Fruits

Blueberries contain polyphenols called anthocyanins, which give them their bright blue color and help boost immunity in our bodies. Blueberries can be eaten fresh or frozen. Add frozen blueberries to a morning smoothie. Add frozen blueberries to pancakes. Add fresh blueberries to chia pudding, gluten-free oatmeal or dairy-free yogurt. Eat them alone as a snack.

Cranberries are acidic in nature and contain proanthocyanidins, which is why they are recommended to treat UTIs (urinary tract infections). The proanthocyanidins act as a barrier to the bad bacteria that is in the bladder or urethra. Cranberries, unfortunately, have added sugar when you buy them as a drink or cook with them. My family loves the cranberry relish I make around the holidays which is chock-full of sugar. If you can tolerate the bitter flavor of raw cranberries or raw cranberry juice, the benefits of reducing bad bacteria is highly beneficial, especially if you are prone to UTI's.

Other berries are especially important to include in our daily diet because of their polyphenol compounds that reduce inflammation in our bodies. Like blueberries, the polyphenols are known as anthocyanins and give berries their bright colors.

Papaya contains an enzyme known as papain, which is used to hydrate and exfoliate the skin by gently removing unwanted dead skin cells. Papaya digests cell proteins internally and externally, and it can also be used topically through a fruit enzyme. Papaya can also be eaten fresh or cooked like a vegetable.

Watermelon contains lycopene which helps to neutralize free radicals. Watermelon also contains choline, which reduces chronic inflammation.

Vegetables

Cruciferous vegetables include broccoli, kale, brussel sprouts, cauliflower, onions, celery and red cabbage. Broccoli contains sulforaphane, which blocks enzymes associated with joint pain and can reduce inflammation in the body caused by sugar or poor diets. Broccoli can be eaten raw with dips, such as hummus or ranch dressing. Dress it up and roast it with a caramelized crunch. It is a colorful addition to pasta dishes and casseroles. My mom always makes the best broccoli. She blanches it in water for one minute, then shocks it in an ice bath. For flavor, she sautés the broccoli with olive oil and garlic, with a sprinkle of Romano cheese.

Dark, leafy green vegetables *contain sulforaphane, which is associated with blocking enzymes that are linked to joint pain and may also be able to prevent or reverse damage to blood vessel linings caused by chronic blood sugar problems and inflammation.*[9]

Vitamin E Major explains, "Vitamin E may play a key role in protecting the body from pro-inflammatory molecules called cytokines—and one of the best sources of this vitamin is dark green veggies. Dark greens and cruciferous vegetables also tend to have higher concentrations of vitamins and minerals—like calcium, iron, and disease-fighting phytochemicals."

Onions contain quercetain, which decreases histamines in the body. *Onions' anti-inflammatory properties have made them a popular home remedy for asthma for centuries.*[9]

Celery is high in vitamin C, which means that it keeps the immune system healthy. It also contains luteolin, a bioflavonoid that reduces free radical damage to cells. Apigenin is also found in celery and is used in Chinese medicine to prevent gout and arthritis. Celery can be eaten raw, added to salads, or served with peanut butter or almond butter with raisins for a healthy kid snack.

Red cabbage is usually prepared in sauerkraut, or cole slaw, or eaten raw. Sauerkraut which is fermented cabbage, is beneficial for the body because the fermentation process creates digestive enzymes. These enzymes help keep the gut healthy and digest the cabbage to boost the body's immunity to ward off illness. Raw cabbage is great for a crunch in salads. High in fiber, it prevents constipation and helps detoxify to remove unwanted toxins from the gut and intestines.

Nuts

Walnuts are high in Omega 3's and contain antioxidants such as L-arginine, alpha-linoleic acid and phenolic antioxidants, thus their ability to reduce pain and inflammation. A walnut-rich diet can even result in prevention of bone loss. Major loves all nuts. *"All nuts are packed with antioxidants, which can help your body fight off and repair the damage caused by inflammation. Nuts (along with fish, leafy greens, and whole grains) are a large staple of the Mediterranean diet, which has been shown to reduce inflammation in as little as six weeks."*[59] Add walnuts to non-dairy yogurt or make a to-go nut mix with walnuts, almonds, pistachios and pecans. Bake walnuts in cookies, brownies or breads.

Seeds

Hemp seeds get a bad rap because they are grown as cannabis, but the actual hemp seed is rich in essential fatty acids, protein, vitamin E and minerals such as phosphorus, potassium, sodium, magnesium, sulphur, calcium, iron and zinc. Hemp seeds are highly beneficial for our bodies and contain essential fatty acids to help our bodies digest protein, prevent the loss of collagen and elastin and prevent heart disease. Hemp seeds can be purchased in powder form for yogurt and smoothies, can be made into a non-gluten oatmeal or baked with it. At the same time, get a healthy boost of energy and keep your heart healthy.

Chia Seeds are also high in Omega 3's and are high in both soluble and non-soluble fiber, antioxidants, protein and minerals. Chia seeds can help to curb hunger due to their high fiber and protein content. Chia seeds can be tossed into smoothies or mixed with dairy-free milk or yogurt to create a pudding for a meal or snack. They take some getting used to at first, but once you are accustomed, they are easy to eat, digest and add to any meal. Try this easy chia seed pudding. Make a large batch and add to mason jars to provide a quick breakfast or snack.

Chia Pudding:
2 cups unsweetened almond, coconut or cashew milk
1/2 cup chia seeds
2 Tbsp. maple syrup (if you don't like sweet, use 1 Tbsp.)
1 Tbsp. brown sugar
1 tsp. cinnamon
1 tsp. vanilla extract

- In medium bowl, whisk together milk, chia seeds, maple syrup, brown sugar, cinnamon and vanilla.
- Cover & refrigerate overnight (or add to 3-4 mason jars for

individual pudding).

- If it ends up being too sweet, add in fresh berries. And for a great crunch, chop up some almonds and pecans (or nuts of choice).

Herbs

Herbs have been used for thousands of years in food or as an herbal concoction for healing.

Ginger is a common ingredient in Asian and Indian dishes, but other cultures have used ginger for its ability to reduce nausea, loss of appetite, pain, and motion sickness, especially in pregnant women. *Ginger is high in phenolic compounds that are known to help relieve gastrointestinal irritation, to stimulate saliva and bile production and to suppress gastric contractions and movements of food and fluids throughout the GI tract.*[11] Ginger can be used in stir-fry dishes, added to soups, steeped to make tea or even a simple syrup.

Turmeric is a relative of ginger and is known for its bright yellow color. It is the main ingredient in most Indian dishes. Turmeric produces an ingredient called curcumin, which is anti-inflammatory and can act like hydrocortisone when applied topically or like Motrin internally. Turmeric can be used in cooking chicken or added to soups for a deeper flavor or coloring, but remember to start out lightly. It is a strong herb with an overpowering flavor. It may take a little getting used to.

Curcumin *Studies have shown that curcumin's anti-inflammatory effects are comparable to the potent drugs hydrocortisone and phenylbutazone and OTC anti-inflammatory agents, such as Motrin.*[12]

Fats

Avocados, olive oil, coconut oil and fatty fish are great sources of good fats. One avocado provides the body with vitamins A, C, E, K & B6 along with an enormous amount of potassium and "healthy fat." Oleic acid is the primary fatty acid in avocados and can lower the risk of heart disease. *Avocados are also rich in Omega 3's and provide all 18 essential amino acids necessary for the body to form a complete protein. Avocado protein is readily absorbed by the body because they also contain fiber.*[13] Chop them up for tacos, salads, or chicken dishes. Freeze them for a morning smoothie, or just eat them whole. Make homemade guacamole and dip cucumbers, carrots, celery and snap peas for a healthy and fun snack.

Fish

Cold-Water Fish are one of the best dietary sources of Omega-3 fatty acids. Our bodies do not produce Omega 3's so we need to take it from dietary sources to continue to survive. *Cold water fish are high in omega 3's because they live in environments that promote production of this fat very well. Eating the right fish can get a high amount of omega-3's into your diet while avoiding dangerous contaminants like mercury. The best fish to eat include salmon, sardines, smelt, shad and anchovies. Tuna and mackerel are particularly known for having high amounts of mercury.*[14] Not all fish are equal, so be sure it is fresh. If fresh is not available, buy frozen. Identify the source of the fish and buy organic or free-range if possible. These fatty fish also help keep the skin hydrated and supple.

The good news is that despite all the bad foods out there, there are plenty of great foods to choose from. Hopefully, this list will help with family meals. While it may seem difficult to switch to a fully-clean lifestyle, I try to stick to the 80/20 rule. As long as my family and I eat well 80% of the time, it's ok to indulge every now and again. Who wants to cook all the time anyway?

DIETS

Diets can be different for everyone. Throughout the years, there have been many diet fads including fat-free, Atkins, South Beach, Paleo, dairy-free, gluten-free or grain-free. Whatever the research, we always come back to the fact that eating a clean diet of plant-based foods, lean meats, seafood and good fats is best to maintain a healthy body and keep our weight under control.

We know that we can exercise like crazy, and we will not lose weight unless we have a proper diet. Even with exercise, we may end up gaining weight because the diet is not balanced. A proper diet supplies the body and organs with the nutrients we need to function and work at maximum capacity. American diets are full of processed foods, sugar, gluten and dairy. A multitude of health problems are increasing, such as autoimmune diseases, diabetes, cancers and even mental-health concerns such as depression.

These days, our lives are so busy. It seems that the easiest thing to do

Samantha's Cleanse

I'm not saying that we should NEVER eat out. I am a mom of three, and some days I just don't feel like cooking or dealing with dishes. For these times, convenience meals and a night out are very enjoyable. It just cannot be our lifestyle. Moderation is key, even with processed foods. With that being said, I do want to talk about what a good diet should look like. Some of you are blessed with children who love their veggies, and they will scream when they are taken away. I am NOT one of those parents. I yearn for the day when my kids will sit at the dinner table without a fight or yell at me because the kitchen smells "yucky" and how they are not eating "a yucky dinner." Ah, someday...

For those with children like mine, consistency is key. Trust me, being consistent does NOT always work, no matter what the parenting books may tell you. At every meal, I make sure EVERY plate has fruit during lunch and at least one vegetable on their plate at dinner. Eating it is the struggle, but it is there, and they see me eating it every single day.

is grab a quick, prepared meal from the grocery store or stop at a fast food restaurant in between shuffling kids from activity to activity or in between deadlines and meetings. Quick meals tend to be processed foods full of hidden ingredients. It is hard to even pronounce the ingredients on the labels, let alone know them. In addition, manufacturers conceal ingredients like wheat, dairy and sugars with alternate names, so we do not actually recognize them in the label.

DIFFERENT DIETS

Finding the right diet can be difficult, but look for one that is sustainable for life and creates a balanced approach. Obviously, eating tons of red meat and no carbs is not sustainable for life. However, when eating well most of the time, carbs and red meats can be included (if there isn't a sensitivity or allergy).

The Mediterranean Diet

Think about changing your life and improving your health by eating foods with family or friends and wine in moderation. The Mediterranean-style diet started the whole "clean eating" trend in America because the Italians eat gluten daily and do not have the intolerance issues we have in America. However, they also eat fresh fish, lots of vegetables and practically drink olive oil with their meals (ok, that's my family). They do cook almost every meal with olive oil, which is a good fat.

Highlights of the Mediterranean Diet
- Encourages an abundance of fruits and vegetables at every meal
- Consumes very few processed foods so their bodies are clean, healthy and full of energy
- Olive oil is the main healthy fat
- Includes moderate to low amounts of cheese or dairy
- Consumes protein from meats or fish high in Omega 3's a few times a week
- Very little red meat is served

Those who live in the Mediterranean region and follow this diet are also highly active people. Physical activity is very important to them, which means that the diet needs to follow their active lifestyles. Consuming processed foods and sugars would not help them live life to the fullest.

The Paleo Diet

Another diet that is healthy and filling is the Paleo Diet. Many people who follow this diet tend to stick with it because there are so many delicious options and meal choices. Some die-hard Paleo fans have discovered mock versions of their favorite desserts, so there is no need for deprivation.

Highlights of the Paleo Diet

- Similar lifestyle to Mediterranean, except consume grass-fed, lean red meats
- Consume fruits and vegetables to keep healthy
- Include good fats from avocados, nuts, seeds and olive oils, providing necessary Omega 3's
- Exclude legumes, such as beans and peas, which can be controversial
- Avoid all grains, processed foods, sugars, gluten and dairy

Gluten-Free & Dairy-Free Diets

Gluten and dairy are highly inflammatory ingredients and are best eliminated from the diet. However, minimizing these two can also activate desirable symptoms.

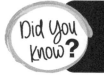 **Did you know?** Even if labels indicate a product is GF or DF, the product can still be manufactured or packaged in a facility that also processes wheat, nuts, dairy or soy, thereby contaminating the food.

Be Aware of Labels and Cross-Contamination

Someone who is highly sensitive to ingredients can have an adverse reaction from eating them, whether they are consumed directly or in contaminated foods during processing.

- While choosing gluten-free (GF) and dairy-free (DF), be sure to carefully read food labels. Manufacturers can hide gluten in gluten-free foods and dairy in dairy-free foods.
- Read labels to make sure the GF or DF product was not manufactured or packaged in a facility that also processes wheat, nuts, dairy or soy.
- When you go out to restaurants, the opportunity for cross-contamination of food products is really high. Most restaurants now offer gluten-free menus. However, be sure to tell the server and chef of any gluten sensitivities to prevent cross-contamination.
- Dairy is less likely to have cross-contamination issues but it can still happen if whey proteins are added to cereals or grains. Read food labels and ask lots of questions.

DETOX

Since many of the foods we eat are highly processed and include gluten, dairy, soy and sugars, some people opt for detox programs. Detox programs aid with digestion, cleansing the gut, promoting gut health and providing healthy and wholesome, nourishing foods via 'clean eating.'

Various programs are on the market and run anywhere from one to thirty days. I have tried many of them, including silly three-day lemon, water and maple syrup fasts; full 30-day regimens that include specific foods, supplements and smoothies; shake programs; and everything in between. I can honestly say that at the end of the program I always feel great, more energetic and my stomach is always flat.

More recently, detox programs include 1-2 smoothies or shakes a day. In addition, supplements, which aid in digestion also cleanse the gut so it can do what it does best; clean itself. Many of the programs now offer specific foods to eat with simple recipes that can be made for your entire family. Most eliminate common allergens such as gluten, dairy, soy and sugar.

Dieticians, chiropractors, functional health or naturopathic doctors can help guide you through the process. A healthy detox works to nourish your body with the right nutrients to rid toxins. Each detox has its own process and its own list of benefits, so it is important to work with a professional medical person to figure out which one will work for you. Recently, the term, "Functional Health," is becoming more common because doctors want to help treat their patients differently with health from the inside, such as detoxes and nutrition.

How Does the Detox work?

Many of the foods in the American diet create inflammation in the body, which stems from the gut. When the intestinal tract is inflamed, eventually microscopic tears appear in the gut. The nutrients then seep out, preventing full absorption of the nutrients needed.

Samantha's Cleanse

I am very Type A, and when I detox, I follow everything to a 'T.' During the process, even though I'm not craving them, I think to myself, 'I'd love a piece of pizza and a bag of dark chocolate almonds.' The actual idea that I can't have it makes me want them more. When I finish the program, I always want to order pizza and buy a bag of dark chocolate almonds. I don't because with all the effort I gave, I don't want to mess it up immediately. The nice thing is that the 'thought craving' isn't too difficult to get past because my pants fit loosely and I feel amazing. But we are all human, and sometimes the bad habits creep back. A few months later, we are back to where we were. In between detoxes, I really have worked hard to eliminate and avoid gluten and dairy. I keep sugars to a minimum. I know these foods are highly inflammatory, and I honestly feel the difference after eating these foods; not to mention, I don't want my acne to return!

A detox program eliminates these foods from your diet so the body can heal and the gut can restore itself during the time of the program. Once the gut is healthy again, it functions properly with increased energy and restored digestion. Since a healthy gut significantly decreases inflammation, the risks for heart disease, diabetes, auto-immune diseases, cancer and even hormone imbalances are decreased. However, after the detox, clean eating must be followed for the detox to decrease such risks. After the detox, some immediate changes occur, including increased energy, clearer skin, less bloating, weight loss, little to no cravings and feeling better.

When Do A Detox?

Some experts suggest that a detox is good to do in the spring and fall. Others recommend right after the holidays because of all the inflammatory foods consumed in during the 6 or 7 weeks. Personally, I like to do mine in the spring. This way, I feel better starting summer without worrying too much about my swimsuit. This past year, I detoxed in January. I am always cold, and when living in Chicago, I was freezing. The two smoothies a day could not keep me warm. Spring and fall work best for me.

I highly recommend doing a detox with someone. Find an accountability partner, and a dietician, naturopath, chiropractor or functional health doctor, especially if you've never done a detox before. These professionals will guide you, offer support and adjust certain elements as needed.

CLEAN EATING

Clean eating is not a trend; rather, it is a lifestyle. Clean eating is preparing and eating wholesome foods, so we function better and stay healthy.

Components of Clean Eating
- Fruits and vegetables are important and should be part of every meal. To be healthy, we need fruits and vegetables to give us

vitamins, antioxidants and minerals for energy.

- Lean meats or seafood, especially grass-fed red meats. Everything in moderation is key, but you want to keep protein in the diet because that's what keeps our bodies full from meal to meal.

Components of Living with Balance

- Everything we consume has calories.
- Everybody needs to eat a certain number of calories daily. If we consume too many calories, we gain weight. When we consume fewer calories, we lose weight.
- A calorie doesn't always equal a calorie. A 100-calorie cookie and a 100-calorie apple will be utilized differently by the body.
- Carbohydrates get a bad rap because of the gluten that is in practically every side dish. However, carbs provide energy. The more activity we perform, the more energy we need, especially post-workout. Choosing the right carbs, like sweet potatoes, can give your body the energy it needs while supplying you with proper nutrition too. The carb-free diet never worked well for people because they all had low energy. Our bodies are designed to eat carbohydrates, just not in the way we currently do.
- Good fats are also important and help keep our bodies full until the next meal. Avocados, olive oil, coconut oil and fatty fish are great sources of good fats.
- Always drink lots of water. Adding lemons to room temperature water helps detoxify and neutralize the body. Most of the foods we eat are acidic and lemons also bring the pH level of your body back to neutral.

Healthy Tip

Try cooking with coconut oil instead of canola, vegetable or olive oil. It isn't as complicated as it seems and there isn't a difference in flavor. Coconut oil can be heated at a higher temperature than olive oil, which is why it is becoming the preferred oil of choice.

Reaching a healthy, balanced lifestyle does not need to be all or nothing. Changing a bad habit or two at a time will ensure a higher success rate. The positive changes will provide motivation to continue healthy living!

SENSITIVITIES & REACTIONS – IT'S INTERNAL!

As we now know, our skin is an organ of our body. Its job is to filter harmful or prevent unhealthy elements from breaking through our skin and entering the systems of our body. It is also a detoxification organ. If any system is off balance or holding too many toxins, the skin acts like an alarm and reacts with various skin conditions.

Samantha's Cleanse

Sugar, truly, is the enemy in the American diet because there is sugar in practically every food we eat. To go truly sugar-free is the most difficult lifestyle change because you literally cannot eat ANYTHING processed. It all must be clean. Sugar is even hidden in sugar-free foods. Hence the importance to read food labels!

SUGAR

Studies have shown that sugar can be more addictive than cocaine! That is a scary thought because most of us do crave sugar or sweets on a regular basis. Those who know me well know that I am a sugar addict and can't go a day without something sweet. I try very hard to keep it out of my house, but somehow its creeps into my shopping cart. It mysteriously manages to find its way into my sugar cabinet (which is hidden from my kids). I am definitely addicted to sugar!

Sugar in Our Bodies

Excess sugar can affect our bodies both internally and externally. High amounts of sugar causes proteins from the body and proteins from the sugars to link together and create Advanced Glycation End Products (AGEs).

Many of us know that the American diet is highly processed and lacks clean foods such as lean proteins, fruits and vegetables. This results in AGEs to form in the body; also, known as *Glycotoxins, are a group of highly oxidant compounds with pathogenic significance in diabetes and several other chronic diseases.*[10] Besides the fact that AGEs are bad for our bodies, they are in all foods, including fruits and vegetables. Cooking these low-AGEs foods can result in new AGEs to form. We obviously cook our meat because we know it is unsafe to eat raw meat. However, the process of roasting, broiling, searing, frying and, especially grilling can speed up the AGEs process. Grilling is the worst way to cook meat because the charred pieces on the meat that we love so much is bad for us and can be potentially carcinogenic.

Samantha's Cleanse

I've tried everything to stop the cravings. Even when I am off sugar for a cleanse, I am constantly thinking of sweets, even if I am not truly craving them. It is a constant challenge to stay strong and not give in to my weak side. I am also aware of the feeling when I crave sugar, like right after any meal. While we were growing up, my mom did not serve dessert every night. That is ironic, since it is now when my cravings strike the strongest. During the day, if I'm busy, I don't think about it. However, when I'm home with the kids, those are the days I tend to give into sweets more often and have several instead of my one-a-day.

Most of you can probably relate because almost every client of mine and all my friends all say the same thing. We have at least one piece of cookie, candy or treat daily. It is not necessarily bad to have a treat, but it is the impact sugar has on our bodies that makes it so bad.

Internally, glycation creates inflammation in our bodies, which can cause a myriad of inflammatory diseases. If we were to just eliminate inflammation from our bodies, we would feel better, reduce chances for food allergies, autoimmune disease and cancer. Our skin would be clear, and we would age more slowly. Inflammation is at the root of all these skin and health conditions. We need to work hard to achieve a healthy diet and lifestyle which includes finding a way to eliminate sugar completely.

Externally, since AGEs are not normal for our bodies, they attack the collagen and elastin proteins in our dermis. Remember, the dermis is responsible for skin elasticity and keeping it smooth and firm. When the dermis is impacted by AGEs, it accelerates the aging process and alters the cell structure and functions. This causes deeper wrinkles and duller, weaker and sagging skin.

Treat the AGEs Skin

When the skin is suffering from glycation, it is usually fragile and compromised because it rapidly slows the skin's cellular turnover rate. However, treating the skin both at home and with an esthetician is possible. Estheticians need to be careful because the skin is compromised, which means that the body most likely is suffering from some sort of disease. Follow these do's and don'ts for the healthiest recovery.

Don't
- Never use any aggressive treatments, such as peels and microdermabrasion.
- Avoid at-home treatments, which include Alpha-Hydroxy acids (AHAs), retinols, aggressive facial scrubs or mechanical scrubbing brushes.

Do
- Use enzymes in the spa or at home to gently remove those unwanted dead skin cells.
- Keep the skin hydrated.
- Focus on hydrating and calming the skin because skin inflammation or reactions to products is extremely likely when you have glycated skin.

- Estheticians can use treatments such as LED light therapy or microcurrent to stimulate the skin while reducing surface inflammation.
- At home treatments, should include:
  - > A gentle cleanser in the morning and evening
  - > An enzyme once a week to keep the skin exfoliating, along with a hydrating moisturizer.
  - > Serums can be used, but the ingredients need to be checked, because you need to avoid AHA's, retinols, and toxic or inflammatory ingredients, such as propylene glycol, fragrances, or parabens.

Furthermore, to truly prevent skin issues and heal the skin, avoid sugars and other inflammatory ingredients. Carefully read labels! Sugars are hidden in food labels, and we see some of the more common ones, such as sucrose, maltose, dextrose, fructose, glucose, etc. If it ends in –ose, it's a sugar. There are many other names for sugars on food labels as well.

Samantha's Story Time

During my work days, my clients are scheduled one after the another. I snack on nuts and protein bars throughout the day to stay energized. One afternoon, I was eating during a break with my son, Zachary.

He said, "Mom, these bars are healthy."

I asked, "Why?"

He replied, "Look, it says 'sugar-free.' Why are they so sweet?"

I responded, "It has sugar in it." He looked at me with a confused expression, which was certainly understandable.

I read the label and sure enough, *sucrose* was on the label. Kids are so smart! He couldn't understand why the label said sugar-free, if there's sugar in the protein bar. Frankly, neither can I.

Hidden Sugars

Many processed foods contain hidden sugars, but the ingredient list may not specifically list 'sugar.' The following list offers some of the most common names. There are many other names that are hidden and not identified as sugar. In addition, manufacturers are starting to group sugars with other ingredients to rename and disguise them.

Labels for Hidden Sugars[15]

Agave Nectar
Barley Malt
Beet Sugar
Brown Rice Syrup,
   Rice Bran Syrup,
   Rice Syrup
Brown Sugar
Buttered Sugar
Buttered Syrup
Cane Juice,
   Cane Juice Crystals or
   Cane Sugar, Evaporated
   Cane Juice
Cane Sugar
Caramel
Carob syrup
Caster Sugar
Coconut Sugar
Confectioner's Sugar
Corn Sweetener,
   Corn Syrup, High Fructose
   Corn Syrup, Corn Syrup
   Solids
Corn Syrup,
   High Fructose Corn Syrup,
   Corn Syrup solids
Crystalline Fructose
Date Sugar
Dehydrated Cane Juice,
   Cane Juice Solids,
   Cane Juice Crystals
Demara Sugar
Dextran
Dextrin or Maltodextrin

Diastatic Malt, Malt Syrup
Diatase, Diatasic Malt
Ethyl Maltol
Fructose
Fruit Juice,
   Fruit Juice Concentrate,
   Dehydrated Fruit Juice,
   Fruit Juice Crystals
Galactose
Glucose
Golden Sugar, Golden Syrup
Golden Syrup
Honey
Invert Sugar
Lactose
Malt Syrup
Maltodextrin
Maltose
Maple Syrup
Molasses or
   Blackstrap Molasses,
   Molasses Syrup
Muscovado Sugar
Oat Syrup
Organic Raw Sugar
Panela, Panocha
Refiners Syrup
Sorghum, Sorghum Syrup
Sucrose
Sugar or Syrup
Tapioca Syrup
Treacle
Turbinado Sugar
Yellow Sugar

Be sure to review the variations of the word 'sugar' in the sugar table to the left. If you are reducing your sugar intake, it is important to know this list.

Gluten and dairy products can also contain sugars. For example, sugar is added to breads, pastas and baked goods. Yogurt is the most commonly consumed food and most brands and flavors are very high in sugar; even the sugar-free ones! The sugar outweighs the probiotic in these foods, and some don't even have high enough amounts of live cultures to make it a true probiotic. This creates a vicious cycle. Awareness and diet changes will help you live a healthier lifestyle.

Kick the Sugar Cravings

I know it is easier said than done, but try to make it a point to reach for fruits or vegetables when a sugar craving hits. Even a handful of almonds can help curb the cravings. Remember, your body is only craving something because it is lacking in something else. Be a little more mindful when you reach for that sugary treat every day. We are all a work in progress!

Healthy Tip

Reach for fruits, vegetables or even a handful of almonds when a sugar craving hits!

CANDIDA

One of the biggest reasons why our skin becomes inflamed or skin conditions show up is that most Americans suffer from candida, which are bad bacteria that live in our gut. *Candida is a genus of yeasts and is the most common cause of fungal infections worldwide. Many species are harmless. However, when mucosal barriers are disrupted or the immune system is compromised, they can invade or cause disease.*[16]

Candida is found in our gut (small and large intestines) and feeds off antibiotics or sugar in our bodies. When we think of gut health and helpful verses harmful bacteria living in our intestines, candida is often overlooked. Candida attacks our immune system, which results in toxic overload, mainly caused by diet. *There are many mental and physical symptoms of candida including migraines, obesity, MS, lupus, depression, endometriosis, athlete's foot, miscarriages, hypothyroidism, acne, rosacea, eczema, and psoriasis.*[17]

When it comes to candida, we have already learned about our biggest culprit, sugar. By now, we understand sugar is consumed in excess by most Americans (myself included). Even though the food may be sugar-free it will contain some form of sugar. Candida loves sugar. The more sugar we eat and crave, the more the candida thrives in our guts. A former boss had shared that her client's skin problems were related to an excess of yeast in the body, also known as candida overgrowth.

There are ways to combat the candida. Reducing sugar is the number one priority. While taking antibiotics, the nurse may suggest yogurt for the probiotic benefits that help keep your digestive tract healthy during the course of antibiotics. In addition, a probiotic may help accelerate the elimination process.

The Candida Diet[18]
by Lisa Richards lists six easy tips to kick your sugar cravings.

1) **Remove sugary foods from the house.** Simple, but how many of us actually follow this step? I certainly don't and my kids are always bringing home candy from birthday parties or school. There might be protests from your family, but you need to explain to them how the sugar has been impacting your health. *If they manage to give up sugar too, you might just be sparing them from future health complications like heart disease or Type 2 Diabetes.*[18]

2) **Find a good substitute.** I remember spending lots of time at my grandparent's house, who were beekeepers. They put honey

on everything, including pancakes. Tasting honey still brings me back to those days of fresh honey on fluffy buttermilk pancakes. *Sweeteners like Stevia or Xylitol are very useful for candida sufferers; they provide a sweet taste without spiking blood sugar. However, to really eliminate your sugar cravings in the long term, you should try to reduce your dependence on sweet-tasting foods altogether.*[18]

3) **Prepare ready-to-eat snacks.** *It's important to have snacks in the house that won't make your Candida worse.*[18] Pick a day of the week for grocery shopping and meal and snack preparation. Chop up veggies and store in baggies for a quick and easy go-to snack. Then when you are crunched for time to make dinner, veggies are already chopped, saving prep-time and a drive-thru run.

4) **Eat Small Meals.** 5-6 small meals throughout the day will keep blood sugar level and prevent feeling too full from eating in a hurry. *If you can manage to regulate your blood sugar levels throughout the day, you will take a big step towards beating your sugar addiction. That's because every spike in blood sugar is followed by a crash.*[18] Many dieticians recommend eating three balanced meals with protein, fruits, vegetables and good fats to satisfy cravings, stabilize blood sugar and stave off hunger until the next meal. Do what works for your body and your schedule.

5) **Plan, Prepare and Be Creative with Meals**
   - Plan meals, snacks and write the grocery list for the week.
   - Plan to cook most nights with lean proteins and lots of vegetables.
   - Schedule the meals and snacks for the week. This will help reduce the temptation for processed meals when you're in a hurry.
   - Shop at the healthiest stores.
   - Prep ingredients for the week on the same day as the shopping.
   - Add lots of herbs and spices to liven up your meals, and you will soon start to enjoy tasty savory foods just as much as sweet dishes.[18]

6) **Take your time.** Sugar can be as addicting as cocaine, so it will take time to make the turn. When eating processed and sugary foods for a long time, *quitting cold turkey is rarely a good idea. You can make your journey to a sugar-free life much more comfortable by gradually reducing your sugar consumption. Start by cutting half the amount of added sugar you eat.*[18] Sometimes, our cravings come from being hungry or not eating enough of the right foods. Start a food journal for one to two weeks. Write down everything you eat, how you feel at the time of eating and note when you crave sugar. This helps identify the amount of food consumed and times of the day you crave sugar. Then you can adjust your diet to distract cravings and eat healthier.

How Candida Affects the Skin

Candida can be a significant factor with those who suffer from acne. Many people have an overload of candida in their gut and do not even realize it. If you are like me who craves sugar no matter the cleanse or lifestyle change, there is most likely an excess of candida in your system. Candida becomes stronger and more abundant with sugar intake. This makes it more difficult to eliminate.

Oftentimes, acne is the result of excess candida along with skin conditions such as rosacea, eczema and psoriasis. Eliminating sugar is the right step. In addition, detoxifying the intestines removes these bacteria, prevents further breeding and reduces the good bacteria or "flora" in our gut.

Teenagers are the most common age group suffering from candida-related acne. Due to their lifestyles and teenage eating habits, acne breakouts are common all over the face and sometimes can result in deep, cystic acne. The most believed common solution is to visit the dermatologist, who prescribes antibiotics. Antibiotics destroy the good bacteria in the gut, which opens the door for candida to breed. If the acne problem is candida-related, antibiotics exacerbate the situation. Dermatologists also prescribe topical treatment, which hides the acne symptoms by weakening the immune system of our skin. Teenagers can see impactful results and clearing of acne with an esthetician who specializes in healthy lifestyle support systems. Acne will clear with a consistent plan including a gentle home skin care schedule, facials, diet changes and a detox. It will take longer than antibiotics and topical treatment plans because it is cleaning from the inside out. However, if you know the health benefits, it is worth it.

Like gaining weight, skin conditions do not happen overnight. It is the result of many months or years of improper diet or poor skin care that one day presents itself on the skin. Most clients try different approaches for several months before seeing a dermatologist or their esthetician for the problem. Prolonging treatment, even inadvertently, just means that it will take time to resolve the issue. Patience and faith in the natural process for about 4-6 weeks will give the time required to notice differences. However, this approach focuses on keeping the skin and body healthy during the entire process.

A food journal helps me identify foods that trigger my clients' skin conditions. After 2-3 weeks of journaling, we adjust home care, diet and add an internal detoxification to help rid the skin of its problems. With the acne problems I had, I know this process works because I followed it. After a detox and embracing a healthier diet, my acne actually cleared in two months.

GLUTEN

Gluten is one of the most controversial foods in the American diet. We will get to the bottom of the myths and explain exactly how gluten impacts our health.

What Is Gluten?

Gluten is a group of proteins found in wheat, rye, barley and possibly, oats. These proteins can trigger a reaction in the immune system causing all types of health issues such as skin conditions and intestinal issues. The American diet consists of a surplus of bread, pasta, sugar, cakes, cookies, crackers, and processed foods, which all contain gluten. *Gluten causes damage to the small intestine, leading to nutritional deficiencies and an increased toxicity in the body*[19] Those with gluten sensitivities are not able to digest the gluten, causing the body to treat it as an infection or bad bacteria. *People with gluten sensitivity cannot digest it effectively. As a result, they absorb partially-digested protein molecules. The immune system treats these molecules as invaders, and as it attacks these invaders, white blood cells release histamine, which increases inflammation. Inflammation increases insulin resistance in nearby cell structures. Insulin resistance leads to blood sugar problems, which is linked to acne.*[19]

When we consume wheat, we add to the inflammation in our gut. Our bodies are not designed to tolerate gluten. When consuming gluten in any form, it passes through our intestines, causing the intestines to expand. Once the gluten has passed through, our intestines shrink and return to their normal size. After many years of expanding and contracting, the intestines develop microscopic tears which cause nutrients and food to filter out into our body. Hence the term, "leaky gut." The only way to fix this is to eliminate gluten from our diet or do a detox. Fortunately, the intestines quickly repair themselves from damage.

Along with sugar, gluten is hidden in our foods and has various names. *The following food additives or processed foods contain gluten:*[20]

Ingredients for Hidden Gluten

Baking Powder *(contains wheat or corn)*
Boullion Cubes or Stock Cubes
Candy that may be dusted with flour
Canned Soups
Caramel Coloring and Flavoring
Cheese Spreads and other processed cheese foods
Chocolate *(may contain malt flavoring)*
Cold Cuts, Wieners, Sausages *(may have gluten to cereal fillers)*
Dextrin
Dip and Dry Sauce Mixes
Dry Roasted Nuts and Honey Roasted Nuts
Extenders and Binders
French Fries in restaurants *(same oil can be used for wheat-containing items)*
Gravies *(check thickening agent or liquid base)*
Honey Hams *(coating)*
Hydrogenated Starch Hydrolysate
Hydrolyzed Plant or Vegetable Protein
Hydroxypropylated Starch
Ice Cream & Frozen Yogurt *(cows are fed grains containing gluten which may explain why many people react to dairy)*
Instant Teas & Coffees *(cereal products used in some formulations)*
Maltodextrin *(wheat or corn-based)*
Maltose
Mayonnaise *(check thickener or grain-based vinegar products)*
Miso
Modified food starch
MSG
Mustard *(powder may contain gluten)*
Natural and Artificial Colors
Natural and Smoke flavors
Non-Dairy Creamer
Oil, frying *(cross-contamination from corn)*
Poultry & Meats *(check flavorings & bastings & ask about meat glue)*
Pregelatinized Starch
Seasonings *(check labels)*
Sour Cream *(may contain modified food starch)*
Soy Sauce
Textured Vegetable Protein
Vegetable Gum or Protein
Vitamin Supplements *(some brands contain grain based ingredients)*

Bottom Line Tips to Monitor Gluten Intake

- Read food labels.
- Take a picture of the list above and keep it in your phone for reference.
- Remember that dairy can contain gluten because the cows are usually fed grains, which is mostly wheat or corn.
- Read product labels on beauty products because some manufacturers add gluten to their ingredient list.
- Gluten is hidden in stamps, envelopes, toothpaste, lipstick, hairspray, shampoo, detergents, pet food, medications, vitamins, lotions, play-dough and makeup.
- When the mother consumes gluten, it is passed on to breast-fed babies.

In 2004, the Food Allergen Labeling and Consumer Protection Act (FALCPA) became law. *This law ensures that there would be clearer labeling of food for the millions of people with food allergies. FALCPA updates the labeling requirements for all food products regulated by the FDA. FALCPA requires that foods are labeled to identify the eight major food allergens. The eight major food allergens are: milk, egg, fish, shellfish, tree nuts, wheat, peanuts and soybeans.*[21] The law also requires that the specific type of food used be on the label. For example, with tree nut allergies, the type of nut must be listed.

Gluten and the Skin

Those who are sensitive to gluten must read labels on beauty products because some manufacturers add gluten to their ingredient list. Since OTC products contain lots of fillers and harmful ingredients to their products, the gluten will penetrate the skin and enter the body. This will result in an increase in skin conditions, such as acne, rosacea, eczema or psoriasis. In addition, the body will still be dealing with toxic overload from gluten entering the bloodstream.

DAIRY

Dairy is another controversial topic when it comes to our diet because dairy is in many of the foods we enjoy. We consume yogurts and cheeses because we grew up believing that we need the proteins and calcium from dairy. Unfortunately, dairy is also being linked to skin conditions and is a root cause of acne. *Interestingly, cow's milk is a complicated and highly specialized food designed to grow a baby cow. Therefore, it contains all kinds of interesting things – basic nutritional building blocks like proteins, fats and carbohydrates, as well as minerals, vitamins and antibodies, growth factors and other substances to stimulate the development of the little cow.*[22]

Dairy is a mucous-forming product. We notice it after our kids have dairy when they are down with a cold or sickness. The stuffiness increases. A few years ago, a trade magazine article discussed a study about dairy and acne. The study examined three groups of teenagers with acne. The first group consumed any kind of milk desired; whole, 2%, skim, etc. The second group only consumed organic milk. The third group was completely dairy-free. The only group that showed improvement in their acne was the third group who eliminated dairy.

Samantha's Cleanse

I can personally attest to the outcome in the third group. As an adult, I had acne, and at the time, it was very difficult to give up dairy. I thought I was choosing healthy snacks when I ate yogurt every day. Once I gave it up, I have never looked back, because my skin improved. Afterwards, I realized how bloated, gassy and uncomfortable my stomach felt when I ate dairy. At the time, I thought it was going to be super-challenging, but there are so many dairy-free options now. For instance, there are many kinds of non-animal milks at the grocery store, including almond, coconut, cashew, and my personal favorite, a combination of coconut & almond milks. I do not recommend soy milk because of its potential to create estrogen in the body.

Dairy Ingredients

Dairy contains three main ingredients. Two proteins are casein and whey and lactose is the sugar. Let's examine how they can cause inflammation and reactions.

1) **Casein** is found in dairy products that have a high protein content, such as milk, yogurt, ice cream and cheese. *These proteins are commonly found in mammalian milk, making up 80% of the proteins in cow's milk and between 20-45% of the proteins in human milk.*[23] Casein is slowly digested by our body.

2) **Whey** holds most of the milk's lactose and antibodies to pass immune protection from mother to baby. Whey is soft, fine and easier to digest.

3) **Lactose** is a sugar found in the milk of cows and humans. Up to the ages of two to five years, babies have lactase which is a special enzyme in the digestive system to break down the sugars for digestion.

Dairy Intolerances

Lactose Intolerance

The good news is that being lactose intolerant, which most adults are, is not dangerous to our health. There are some dairy products that do not contain lactose, such as heavy cream, sour cream, hard cheeses, butter and ghee.

Lactose is present in all milk, even milk from our mothers. When we are babies, an enzyme called lactase, helps digest mother's milk. *Lactase is usually produced in the intestines. It breaks the lactose down into glucose so the body can absorb it. When the lactose is not broken down into glucose, several things happen. The lactose itself interferes with the normal absorption of water from the food in the intestine – in fact it reverses the process, putting more water into the intestines.*[24]

As cow's milk is added to the daily diet, around the age of one-year-old, babies still produce lactase. Many produce a small amount of lactase even into adulthood. When some systems stop producing lactase altogether, those people become lactose intolerant. The reason being, that cows produce rennet to help their bodies digest their mother's milk. Humans do not produce rennet, which tends to cause digestion problems after consuming dairy. Even when it is fine for you to drink milk or consume dairy, think about your body and how it feels after consuming cheese or yogurt. Are you bloated and gassy? If so, this can be a sensitivity to dairy.

Once our body stops producing lactase, our bodies are no longer able to digest dairy from a cow. We have seen dairy allergies for several years. This is not a new discovery, like gluten. The lactose-intolerance is more common now because it was finally figured out that dairy is the cause of many digestive complications and issues such as irritable bowel syndrome (IBS), constipation or diarrhea.

Casein

Casein are thick, sticky, clump together and tend to be harder to digest than whey. As previously mentioned, rennet is an enzyme produced in the cow's stomach that helps the baby cows digest their mother's milk. It also breaks down the protein in our systems. The key component in rennet is the enzyme called chymosin. This enzyme is also responsible for curdling the casein in milk and is used to separate milk into curds for cheese. Rennet also contains two other important enzymes, pepsin and lipase. Pepsin breaks down proteins and is responsible for helping the body to digest the dairy in the stomach. Lipase is essential to digestion by helping to break down the fats in the milk.

Whey

Whey is the watery part of the milk, and the proteins are softer, finer and easily digestible. The composition of whey varies depending on the source. When we think of whey, oftentimes, we think of protein powder because of its high nutritional value. Whey is the protein that contains lactose. It is difficult to find proper evidence on this topic because sources vary on whether whey contains more or less lactose than other proteins.

Dairy Allergy vs. Intolerance

There is a definitive difference between a dairy allergy and a dairy intolerance. Each present differently.

Is it a Dairy Allergy?

If someone is allergic to dairy, that condition is not the same as being lactose intolerant.

Dairy intolerance, or sensitivity, means that there isn't enough of the lactase enzyme in the body to break down the lactose (the sugar in dairy). Lactose intolerance is a reaction to either the casein or whey proteins, or possibly both.

A dairy allergy means that an allergic reaction happened because someone is reacting to the protein in milk or dairy. A true allergy results in swelling, hives, rash, flushing, wheezing and oral symptoms such as burning or itching in the throat.

In children, constipation is the most common symptom of a dairy allergy. *Other clues include: eczema, asthma, rhinitis (swollen/itchy nose and eyes), reflux, vomiting, and rectal bleeding.*[23] Some babies are allergic to dairy and their nursing mother must eliminate dairy so she does not pass it on.

Allergy tests performed by allergists will provide definite answers to specific allergies.

Is It a Sensitivity to Dairy?

A dairy sensitivity is the majority of dairy problems in adults. It is not life-threatening, and dairy can still be consumed. Symptoms to sensitivities can include bloating, gas, diarrhea, constipation, bad breath or even heartburn. Unfortunately, there is no way to test for sensitivities. However, eliminate dairy for two weeks to identify changes in digestion. If you feel less bloated, gassy and digestion is working better, you are sensitive. In addition, some dairy consumption can cause skin conditions, such as acne, rosacea, eczema or psoriasis.

Alternatives to Dairy Products

Non-dairy products, such as almond, rice, coconut, and cashew milks, do not contain dairy. They are extracted by breaking down the ingredient they are using to form a liquid. Unfortunately, these are considered processed and lots of sugar and additives are added to make the consistency look, taste and feel like milk.

However, these non-dairy products are a great alternative to cereal, smoothies or protein shakes and chia puddings. There is even non-dairy yogurt for those quick, easy snacks in the middle of the day. Many people want to give up dairy but are worried that they will miss it. Fortunately, we now have plenty of alternatives with these non-dairy products.

I don't recommend consuming large amounts of these products because they are processed and do have sugar added, but to wean yourself off dairy, they are a great way to start.

Chapter 5:
External Factors Influencing Skin Conditions

STRESS

Stress is common in all our lives. For some reason, society dictates that we must constantly be in motion. For some, it is a matter of keeping up with the Jones' because we don't want to miss out or feel behind the times. It is not surprising to know that we create this ourselves. Unfortunately, this lifestyle brings all types of stress into our lives, and many of us do not know how to reduce it, or even manage it. When was the last time you weren't stressed?

This chapter focuses on the impact stress has inside our bodies and outside on our skin. I will share my daily de-stressing tips, hoping that it may help you make your days a little easier.

What is Stress?

Stress is your body's way of responding to any kind of demand or threat. When you feel threatened, your nervous system responds by releasing a flood of stress hormones, including adrenaline and cortisol, which rouse the body for emergency action. On a more positive note, when stress is within your comfort zone, it can help you to stay focused, energetic and alert. Stress is what keeps you on your toes during a presentation at work, sharpens your concentration when you're attempting the game-winning free throw or drives you to study for an exam when you'd rather be watching TV.[25]

According to the Mayo Clinic, *stress symptoms can affect your body, thoughts, feelings, and behavior. Stress that's left unchecked can contribute to health problems, such as high blood pressure, heart disease, obesity and diabetes.*[26]

Stress affects our lives in more ways than we think. We can blame our diets for the way we feel, but stress can have the same impact or worsen the problem. Symptoms such as dull afternoon headaches, insomnia, decreased productivity or fogginess in the brain (such as forgetting to schedule an activity or double scheduling ourselves or our kids) is all linked to stress.

We snap at our family when we feel stressed out and can even feel depressed or blah about life. These are all results of stress. When we are stressed it can lead to health problems, and it also affects our skin.

Stress and the Skin

Did you have that lovely, juicy zit pop up on prom or your wedding day? That was stress from planning and preparing for the most important days of our lives. Let's examine why that happens.

Stress has a negative effect on our skin and the barrier function because it causes our skin to lose water. Losing water is called Transepidermal Water Loss (TEWL), which means that the skin is now susceptible to injury or trauma. TEWL is caused by compromising the skin's barrier which leads to dry skin. During this condition, rosacea or acne breakouts worsen because our bodies are producing the stress hormone, cortisol. When cortisol is increased, it instigates the 'fight or flight' mode within our system. Once activated, we crave sweets, carbs and processed foods. This leads our digestion to become sluggish which can show up in the form of acne, and red bumps or an increased redness from the capillaries that presents itself as rosacea.

The term, "dry skin" is used frequently with different meanings. When

TEWL occurs, the skin lacks the protective layer on the skin's barrier. The skin then begins to look tight or dull and the wrinkles look worse because the skin is dry and has no moisture to keep it hydrated. Once this happens, the skin has become dehydrated (defined below). TEWL prevents the skin from absorbing moisture to keep healthy. Skin needs to have some natural oil to prevent moisture from evaporating. When suffering from TEWL, oil cannot completely solve the problem. However, it does help create a protective barrier until the skin can hold water on its own while the skin repairs itself.

DEHYDRATION VS. DRY SKIN

People use dehydrated and dry skin interchangeably when, in truth, they are individual conditions. They both present in the same manner, so it is difficult to distinguish each one. This makes treatment difficult when trying to combat this skin condition at home. Dehydrated skin reacts differently to care than dry skin. It is important to have treatment and at home products, which will rehydrate, nourish and repair the skin and its barrier.

Dehydration is a man-made skin condition that has a direct relationship to the water content of the skin. The water content can be dry in the epidermis, the dermis or even both. Epidermal dehydration shows up as crepe skin (like crepe paper) or small lines that form when you touch your skin or apply product. *Dermal dehydration causes depletion of the dermis and will ultimately result in deeper wrinkles that are visible on the surface of the skin as well as elastosis and sagging skin.*[27]

Dry Skin

Dry skin tends to feel tight with the need to reapply moisturizer throughout the day. People with dry skin have minimal oil production, have a small number of pores or do not have any enlarged pores. Those who suffer from dry skin need to be careful which products are used so as not to develop dehydrated skin. Switch to a creamy cleanser that doesn't have skin irritants.

Causes for Dry Skin

- Born with it or genetics
- Develops during the aging process
- Processed foods, sugars and food allergens that cause our bodies to be affected by holding in toxins and creating the potential for disease.
- The environment creates TEWL with harsh elements such as wind, dry air, extreme temperatures and pollution.

Dehydrated Skin

Dehydrated skin or Transepidermal Water Loss (TEWL) is more complicated than just dry skin. Recognizing TEWL includes symptoms such as when the skin is normally oily, but suddenly becomes dry; or the oil is noticeable on the face, but feels rough, tight and dry to the touch. It has a very distinct texture because when the barrier becomes compromised, it prevents moisture from being absorbed by the skin.

Dehydrated skin/TEWL is caused by:

1) using the wrong products on your skin.
2) exfoliating too much or using harsh products that strip your skin of oil.
3) the skin's barrier becomes compromised; impairing the barrier and preventing it from holding in or absorbing from moisturizers.
4) increased oil production to compensate for the lack of moisture on the skin.
5) following diets with processed foods, sugars and food allergens.
6) the harsh elements of the environment such as wind, dry air, extreme temperatures and pollution.

Once the skin's barrier becomes compromised, it is difficult to repair, but with the use of proper products, your skin can be repaired.

Caring for Dehydrated Skin

Whether it is dry or dehydrated skin, treating it properly is important. Working with an esthetician can provide facial and home care programs that are adjusted each season with calming and hydrating ingredients to ensure your skin continuously stays hydrated while repairing the barrier.

Steps to Care for Dehydrated Skin

1) Avoid harsh OTC products, physician-grade products or salespeople who are selling product lines without any knowledge of the skin.
2) Use an enzyme exfoliant once a week. It sounds counterproductive to exfoliate while skin's barrier is already compromised, but it's the opposite, because it will prevent the build-up of dead skin cells. Exfoliating helps to absorb serums and moisturizers.
3) Order a customized serum to nourish and rehydrate the skin for your specific needs. The serum contains ingredients that calm, hydrate and soothe the skin. Massage is important because it stimulates circulation, which helps your skin absorb ingredients that will target the cells at the dermal/epidermal junction. This will restore hydration and nourish the skin.
4) Depending on the severity of the skin, apply a facial oil to increase hydration and restore the condition of the oil glands. Not all oil is created equal; there are several oils that can clog the pores. Avoid oil blends, because hidden ingredients may be added into the "blend" and they may be comedogenic (pore-clogging).
5) Keep the skin hydrated with moisturizers.

Five Tips to Hydrate

Here are five tips to help us restore moisture balance in our skin:

Skin Hydration Tip #1 - Moisturizers:

1) Apply your moisturizer both morning and night after cleansing your skin.
2) In the morning, use a moisturizing SPF and a night cream at night. If the SPF moisturizer is not hydrating enough, add a bit of night cream or 100% natural facial oil both morning and night to boost the hydration in your skin. Mix it with the moisturizer or apply over the moisturizer.
3) Beware, some facial oils can be comedogenic, such as avocado, grapeseed or almond oils. OTC products may contain fillers.

Comedogenic products may clog the oil glands and trap dirt and oil in the pore, creating blackheads. Look for professional products that are 100% oil, such as rosehip, jojoba, sesame and sunflower oils. These are the best options for rehydrating.

4) After showering, moisturize immediately and dab your skin dry. Do not completely dry. It is easier to apply moisturizer to damp skin. The quicker you moisturize after your shower, the less time your skin must dry out, and the oil glands won't lose oil production. If your skin feels tight and itchy after you shower, it needs to be hydrated. Keep your body moisturizer in the bathroom, as it is more convenient.

5) Add 100% oil to your body moisturizer, especially on the areas that tend to be dry, like the feet, knees and hands.

Skin Hydration Tip #2 - Cleansers & Toners:

1) Avoid harsh cleansers and irritating ingredients, such as sodium lauryl sulfate/sulfite, propylene glycol, or any products that contain alcohols. If the cleanser is too harsh, skin will feel "squeaky clean" after washing. If it does, your cleanser is stripping your skin of oil and may create dehydrated skin.

2) Do not use toners! Most toners contain alcohol or witch hazel, which dry out the skin. Professional cleansers are pH-balanced and are designed to work with your skin. For this reason, toners are no longer required to neutralize the skin's pH levels. If a line is promoting toners, the pH level of your skin may decrease, which can lead to TEWL.

Skin Hydration Tip #3 - Fragrances & Oils:

1) Avoid any product with fragrances. Fragrances can be made with over 4,000 ingredients. At least 2,000 fragrance ingredients are known allergens or irritants. The FDA does not regulate fragrance ingredients. Some manufacturers hide ingredients such as phthalates and call it a fragrance.

2) Consider how you personally respond to smelling perfume, beauty products, candles or wall fragrances. Do you get a headache? Does it burn your nose and/or cause you to sneeze? Does the smell

bother you? Does it seem strong and overpowering? If you answer "yes," these are irritating fragrance ingredients and should be avoided. Essential oils are made from the actual plant, but can also be irritating to certain skins. Use caution with certain essential oil products.

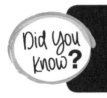

Our hands and feet do not have oil glands, which means they absorb the water differently than the rest of the skin on our bodies. This is why our hands and feet wrinkle and prune when submerged in water for any period of time.

Skin Hydration Tip #4 - Baths & Showers:

1) Do not bathe more than once a day. If you are an avid exerciser, wait until after you exercise to shower. If you exercise later in the day or after work, count that as your daily shower or bath. Americans are the cleanest society, compared to other countries that bathe less often. Many Americans shower twice a day or more. The more you expose your skin to water, the harder it is to keep it hydrated because of the chemicals and minerals in the water.

2) Always shower and bathe in lukewarm water. This is important, especially in the winter months when we are exposed to cold, dry air. The hot temperature from the water dries the skin because heat strips the skin of oil. If you have dry or sensitive skin, make sure the water temperature is warm, but not hot.

3) Limit your time in the shower or bath to 15 minutes. Also, do not run the water continuously. Dry skin develops after 15 minutes because of the exposure to chemicals and minerals in the water.

4) Add a cup of Epsom salt to the water which will stimulate circulation and the lymphatic system. This helps the body release toxins and soothe sore muscles.

Skin Hydration Tip #5 - Clothing:

1) Wear protective clothing when outdoors in all seasons. In the winter when the weather is cold, the wind will chap your delicate

skin. Wind burn creates skin sensitivity, irritation or a burning sensation when applying products.

2) Wear a scarf over your face to protect the skin from the harsh elements. We lived 3 blocks from my son's grade school and unless it was below zero, we walked. I do not ever like to be cold, so I am that crazy over-bundled person who walked to school every day. However, my skin didn't get chapped!

To combat windburn, apply an oil-based moisturizer on the skin before heading outdoors. You still need your protective clothing covering most of your face if it's extremely cold and windy. An oil-based moisturizer creates a mild barrier on your skin to minimize the effects of chapping.

I hope you found these tips helpful and use them daily. Dry skin is such a concern for many people. If I can give a few tips to help you feel less dry, then I've done my job.

STRESS AND THE BODY

The body shows stress in many ways. It changes systems in our body such as hormones, organs and neurological systems. It even alters moods and behavior. Our body responds to stress with many symptoms including frequent headaches, muscle tension, nausea, fatigue, insomnia, and upset stomachs. There are many options to de-stress from the day's events.

Physical Symptoms of Stress[28]

- Low Energy
- Headaches
- Upset stomach including diarrhea, constipation or nausea
- Aches, pain and muscle tension
- Chest pain and rapid heartbeat

- Insomnia
- Frequent colds & infections
- Loss of sexual desire or ability to perform
- Nervousness, shaking, ringing in ear
- Cold or sweaty hands & feet
- Excess sweating
- Dry mouth and difficulty swallowing
- Clenched jaw & grinding teeth

Mood Changes from Stress

- Anxiety
- Panic attacks occur from the constant motion of fight or flight.
- Irritability
- Anger: I know when I'm under stress because I snap and scream at my kids.
- Depression
- Lack of motivation
- Brain fog: We can't remember simple instructions. I'm not one to lose my car keys, but I forget important items at the store, even though it's on my list. I double schedule things because I have too many calendars and forget to add something to the family calendar.

Behavior Changes from Stress

- Eating
- Making unhealthy choices, such as sweet snacks, extra alcohol, carb overload

We have all been in stressful situations throughout our lifetime; it's part of human nature. Behavior can also lead us to start drinking alcohol every night or turn to drugs to help us "feel better." Unfortunately, these are short-lived solutions and once the high wears off, we are back to feeling stressed. Some even become socially withdrawn and avoid events because they do not want to go out, or they just want to stay home and relax. This is fine on occasion, but if this becomes a regular occurrence, then there is a problem and you need to get your stress under control.

DESTRESS TIPS

Now comes the fun part. How can we reduce stress in our lives? There is a lot we can do at home without spending money. These are some simple and easy daily activities that instill calmness.

1) Yoga

Get up an extra 10 minutes earlier every morning. There are many 5 or 10-minute yoga stretch videos on YouTube. You can also join a yoga studio. Just get your body moving. Yoga is great because the intention is set before the class, everyone clears the mind and moves the body. Movement is highly beneficial because it stimulates the circulation flow, stretches muscles, and allows the body to release toxins.

2) Gratitude Journal

Keep a small journal by your bed. Each night, write three things from the day for which you are grateful. Instead of the same three every day, challenge yourself to find something different. You will be surprised how much better you feel about life when you stop to appreciate the small things.

3) Meditation

This may seem daunting. YouTube has a ton of great meditation videos that are as short as 10 minutes. There are choices for either guided meditation or instrumental meditation music. With headphones, meditation will travel. Listen to it in the morning, at lunch, after work, before bed. When you listen to it before sleep, you will be surprised how easy it is to fall asleep when your mind is cleared from the stress of the day. Personally, I like the music-only meditation because I like to fall asleep instead of listening to the entire meditation. However, if you are feeling really stressed, start with a 10 or 15-minute guided meditation to clear your mind.

Guided Meditations
- Deepak Chopra: https://youtu.be/Uin2q_hEHlU
- Yoga Nidra for sleep: https://youtu.be/nod85a5qpSg

- Paul Santisi – Good Night Deep REM sleep:
  https://youtu.be/8KzrrgIpHa8

Music Meditations:
- Sleep Music- Tibetan Singing Bowls:
  https://youtu.be/qIsfwOIzkkQ
- Sleep Music Delta Waves (Deep Sleep):
  https://youtu.be/xQ6xgDI7Whc
- Positive Thinking- Relaxation meditation:
  https://youtu.be/n17BzBecv8w

4) Exercise

A little exercise such as a quick walk around the block, an exercise class or a run will destress you immediately. Most importantly, find a workout that you enjoy which you will be more likely to stick with it. Explore different classes and gyms in your area. If you are not someone who exercises regularly, just start with 1-2 times a week and go at your own pace. Exercise does not have to be competitive, nor a chore. Think of it as medicine to increase health, reduce stress and feel better. The key is to be sure it makes you feel better and does not add stress. Exercise elevates the heart rate, stimulates circulation, increases energy, and releases toxins from the body through sweat. It benefits the whole body internally and externally.

Sometimes we have to force ourselves to try something new, but once you make a change, your stress levels, body and skin will thank you.

SLEEP

Sleep has to be one of my favorite things to do! You would never know it because most days, I'm up at 5:00 a.m. I am usually on the go until 10:00 p.m., when I crash. One of the biggest struggles I had was when my kids were babies, and I was up multiple times a night. I do not do well with interrupted sleep.

There are many things in our lives that either interrupt our sleep patterns or prevent us from falling and staying asleep. This can result in chronic exhaustion, health problems or irritability because our bodies are not getting recharged as necessary.

Sleep is very important because the body shuts down, the brain recharges and organs repair themselves. We need a minimum of eight hours of sleep per night. When we are not getting adequate sleep, our bodies cannot go into repair and refresh mode. This can result in a host of future health problems.

What Happens When We Sleep?

When we sleep, our bodies go through a Circadian Rhythm, which is a 24-hour cycle in the human body that responds to when our environment is light and dark. Melatonin is the hormone secreted by the pineal gland and our brain maintains our circadian rhythm in our bodies during each 24-hour period. Exposure to light especially at night suppresses melatonin and alters circadian rhythm. Depending on how sensitive we are, even a dim light when reading in bed can alter our melatonin production.

Circadian Rhythms can influence sleep-wake cycles, hormone release, body temperature and other important bodily functions. They have been linked to various sleep disorders such as insomnia. Abnormal Circadian Rhythms have also been associated with obesity, diabetes, depression, bipolar disorder, and seasonal affective disorder.[29]

Darkness tells our bodies that it's time to shut down and get ready for sleep. Our brain triggers our body to start to relax, so it can prepare for a good night of sleep for recharging and repairing. Light tells our bodies that it is time to awake and be alert. The brain senses the light, and we begin to awaken. Think about when we turn our clocks back in the fall, we tend to feel exhausted by 6pm because our bodies are not used to that one-hour time change.

Advantages of Sleep

Did you know that we are supposed to spend one-third of our day sleeping? Throughout the course of a night, our body experiences five stages of sleep.

Five Stages of Sleep[30]

Stage 1: Light Sleep
We drift in and out of sleep, easily awakened. If we wake from Stage 1, we remember our dreams.

Stage 2: Shortest Sleep
Eye movements stop, and brain waves become slower.

Stage 3: Deep Sleep*
Extremely slow brain waves, called delta waves, begin to appear. These delta waves are interspersed with similar, faster waves.

Stage 4: Deep Sleep*
Brain produces delta waves almost exclusively.

Stage 5: REM Sleep**
Breathing becomes more rapid, irregular, and shallow. Our heart rate increases and blood pressure rises.

  * During stages 3 and 4 it is very difficult to wake someone, because this is deep sleep.

** Rapid Eye Movement (REM) sleep is the most important stage of sleeping we need in order to feel well-rested in the morning. Many people are not spending a lot of time in REM sleep, which impacts our functionality throughout the day.

When We Sleep
- Brains repair the cognitive function. Without enough sleep, this function is not properly repaired, leaving us to feel sluggish, suffer from brain fog or as if we over-consumed alcohol.

- Organs repair and rejuvenate themselves.
- The body enters fasting mode. When we sleep, our body requires a certain amount of energy and it uses up the glucose we have stored in our body. The glucose is important in helping to release energy for muscle contractions, nerves and regulates body temperature. For effective fasting, it is important to eat the last meal at least two to three hours before bed. When we eat too late, it prevents the fasting cycle to begin and finish as needed. Do you ever wake up feeling horrible during the night? It is most likely because the body is trying to digest food recently consumed. Even worse is when the fast is interrupted by waking and eating or drinking caffeine. Either way, eating too late or eating too early can lead to obesity and weight gain.

Blue Lights

Since the influx of smart phones and tablets, where we have the world at our fingertips, we have a difficult time shutting devices off to unwind at the end of the night. Bright lights or too little light can disrupt our melatonin production. Unfortunately, tablets, phones and TV give off a blue light that stimulates the brain and prevents the brain from a natural shut down.

There are three types of lights that impact the circadian rhythm.

1) Blue lights are emitted from electronic devices. *Blue lights are important during the day, because they boost mood and attention. However, we do know that exposure to [blue] light suppresses the secretion of melatonin, a hormone that alters our circadian rhythm. Even dim light can interfere with a person's circadian rhythm and melatonin secretion.*[31]

Blue lights prevent a proper melatonin release which is why it is difficult to fall asleep or stay asleep at night. A Harvard study compared the effects of exposure of comparable brightness between blue lights and green lights. The finding showed that the *blue light suppressed melatonin for about twice as long as the green light and shifted circadian rhythms by twice as much time.*[31] That is a significantly distinctive disturbance to our night time sleep.

There are blue light-blocking glasses on the market, however, they are primarily designed for night-shift workers, not TV viewers. *Study after study has linked working the night shift and exposure to light at night to several types of cancer (breast, prostate), diabetes, heart disease, and obesity.*[31]

2) Green lights are found to impact our sleep cycles by stimulating our non-visual responses at night. Researchers observed 52 volunteers for a 9-day study to test to see how both blue & green lights affect us at night. *At the start of the light exposure or when exposed to dim light, green light was equally as effective as blue light at stimulating these non-visual effects, but then the effects [of the green light] died off more quickly over time.*[32]

3) Red lights result in less stimulation and are least likely to alter melatonin production.

Advice for Restful Sleep
- Turn off all electronic devices 1-2 hours before bed.
- Avoid caffeine and alcohol for 6 hours before bed.
- Switch night lights to a red light.
- Expose yourself to lots of bright lights during the day.

Disadvantages of Watching TV Before Bed
Before bedtime, many people watch TV until they are ready to fall asleep. Some sit for 3-4 hours. What happens when you do finally head to bed? If this is you, are you able to just lay down and drift to sleep; or are you thinking about the next episode or the list for the next day? Do you ever find yourself dreaming about the show you watched prior to bed? If so, this is a typical occurrence when we watch TV right before bed without proper time to shut down. It happens because the stimulation from the show and the TV light stimulates the brain, which needs time to shut down before falling asleep.

The Vicious Cycle of TV Before the Shut Down Process

1) Watch a stimulating TV show, and the brain cannot turn off.

2) The blue light from the TV told your brain that it is not night time and can't shut down.

3) Go to bed late from watching TV, but end up tossing and turning for another hour before falling asleep.

4) Dream about your show, have horrible nightmares or find that you are actually in the show, only to wake up exhausted and not refreshed at all.

Samantha's Cleanse

I try to read every night before bed. So far, I am still old-school and prefer a book over my tablet. I have felt the difference between the state of reading a paper book verses a tablet reader. With the paper book, my body shifts into a relaxed state quicker. With the tablet, I'm more wired and feel like I need more time to let my body relax.

Sleep and Skin

Lastly, the skin. Did you really think I was going to forget about the skin? When we sleep, our skin, which is also an organ, goes into repair mode. During this mode, collagen and elastin fibers are restored. When the fibers are restored, new skin cells are created, and the skin fights to stay hydrated. Also, damage caused from the day is restored. Over-exfoliating, sun damage, improper products, lack of hydration all contribute to skin's aging process. While we sleep, the skin works to fix the problems created that day, so it can restore it as it was at the beginning of the day.

Hence, the extreme importance to use good product to properly cleanse, treat (with serums) and moisturize prior to bed. Following this process and sleeping 8 restful hours will ensure our skin looks as great as we feel when we wake up the next morning.

EXERCISE

We all know the importance of exercise to maintain proper weight, keep us healthy and feel great. Exercise is important for our skin too! Exercise releases feel-good endorphins, which is why we feel so great after a workout. Exercise along with a proper diet is key to maintain weight or prevent weight gain. Lastly, exercise keeps us healthy because it forces our heart to pump blood and improve our body's circulation. This keeps the circulatory system functioning well, and the lymphatic system removing toxins. These two systems keep the skin healthy by increasing blood flow to the skin, and by releasing toxins through sweat glands.

The most important thing about exercise is to find a workout program that fits your lifestyle and is enjoyable. If you do not like it or it does not fit your lifestyle, you are not going to stick with it. We all have our days and weeks that we fall off the exercise-wagon, but if you enjoy exercise, you are more likely to jump back on after that bump in our life has ended.

What is Exercise?

The physical benefits from exercise are well known in almost every magazine, media, newspaper, TV show, etc. Exercise is very important to maintain health and prevent disease. Exercise is any activity that requires physical effort. Exercise can be as simple as a bike ride, a family walk, a power walk with a friend or as intense as a boot camp or marathon training. The good news - there is an exercise program that will work for you; all you have to do is start!

Benefits of Exercise

The Mayo Clinic shows that there are seven ways that exercise can improve your life.[33]

1) Weight Control

Physical activity burns calories. The more intense the activity, the more calories burned. Workouts can be done at once or broken into short ten-minute activities throughout the day. Both types of workouts still burn calories.

2) Combats health conditions and diseases

Exercise keeps the blood moving smoothly, which decreases your risk of cardiovascular diseases, stroke, metabolic syndrome, type-2 diabetes, depression, arthritis and certain types of cancer.

3) Improves your mood

Physical activity stimulates various brain chemicals that increase happiness and relaxation. It also improves self-esteem and confidence.

4) Boosts energy

Regular exercise, 3-5 days per week, improves muscle strength and boosts endurance by delivering oxygen and nutrients to your tissues. In addition, it promotes the cardiovascular system to work more efficiently, increasing energy.

5) Promotes better sleep

Regular activity aids in falling asleep faster and experiencing a deeper sleep. Be cautious of working out too close to bedtime, as it may keep you awake.

6) Puts the spark back into your sex life

Exercise can leave you feeling energized and looking better, which will have a positive effect on your sex life.

7) Add Some Fun to Life

Unwind, enjoy the outdoors or engage in activities that make you happy. Add movement to your social settings or with family activities. 5Ks with family promote reaching a goal together. Exercise classes with friends allow you to catch up and spend that precious limited time together. Find an activity you enjoy. When you get bored, switch to something new!

Types of Exercise

At the age of 3, my mom enrolled me in ballet, and dance became my life for 20 years. Exercise was ingrained in me at an early point in life, and since then, I have engaged in some sort of physical activity after dance. Before I opened my spa, I spent a few years teaching group fitness classes because I love the class setting. In recent years, I started running, probably to outrun, I mean, chase my children.

Exercise Options

There are countless fitness options at all levels, so everyone can start somewhere. We have all been the new girl or guy who struggled to get through that first class. A great gym or a great instructor will help guide you and offer modifications to help you get through the first few classes until you gain strength to keep up with the rest of the class. Pick a comfortable fitness level, skill set and exercise that you enjoy.

- **Just starting out?**
  Visit local gyms or studios for a test drive. Find one that offers a variety of classes such as swimming, yoga, Pilates, a track for walking or running, personal training, and group fitness classes. Many studios offer free trials or the first week free, which is great to try all the services before committing to the monthly membership fees.

- **Looking for something new with people?**
  Try Zumba, aerobic classes, group training, or spin.

- **Need something faster with a higher calorie burn?**
  Runners have a league of their own that offers great friendships and plenty of groups to help stay consistent with a new running routine. Visit a local running store for running clubs, proper gear, and training advice.

- **Need something advanced?**
  Train for a 5K, 10K, half-marathon, full-marathon, up your game with some more weights, do interval training, cross-fit, flip tires.

- As Nike says, "Just Do It!"

The most important thing to remember is that we all had to start somewhere. Don't be intimidated, just join and have fun with it!

Exercise and the Skin

The greatest benefit skin receives from exercise is the circulation. When we exercise, our blood flow increases, and our body temperature rises. This increase in body temperature tells the hypothalamus, which regulates body temperature, to start cooling so as not to overheat. The increased blood flow supplies the skin with oxygen and vital nutrients to help keep the skin hydrated and functioning properly. Through sweating, it also helps remove waste, such as environmental toxins, harmful ingredients from our beauty products and free radicals from the working cells.

The Sweaty Benefits

Sweat offers many benefits for our skin and bodies:
- protects from overheating, as is a natural air conditioner;
- opens pores to release toxins through special glands, called sudoriferous glands, that are connected to the pores. Sweat is literally just water and does not smell. When the water from the glands mixes with the bacteria on our skin, it produces body odor.

Post-Exercise Skin Care

Exercise is beneficial for our bodies and skin. Sweating is vital to help cool down, and emit toxins from our bodies through sweat. If these toxins sit on the skin for an extended period, they mix with dirt, oil and other environmental toxins, which can result in a breakout. If you don't wash your face regularly after exercising, you will find little white bumps on the forehead or hairline. This happens because after exercise, it is easy to fall into the pattern of running errands or getting too busy with work and the kids before showering (if at all).

Samantha's Cleanse

The best practice after a workout is to shower right away. That doesn't always happen because we are busy and have many tasks to accomplish each day. I used to be guilty of this. My skin was a mess until I finally switched my exercise routine, so I could fit in the shower. A workout at 5:30 a.m. isn't ideal for everyone. However, once I started it, my skin cleared up, and I had extra time in my day because I was already showered and ready to take it on.

Not Going Home After the Workout?

Keep baby wipes in your car or gym bag and occasionally use them. If you are not able to shower after your workout, then bring your cleanser to at least wash your face. Note the recommendation for baby wipes because facial cleansing cloths contain irritating ingredients, fillers and preservatives that are not ideal for your skin. They can cause more harm than good when you use them on a daily basis.

Sweating It Out Dries It Out

Leaving sweat on your skin can dry it out because sweat contains salt, which is drying. Think about how thirsty you feel after eating a salty meal. Salt has the same effect on the skin. If you tend to be dry, wash your face within 20 minutes after working out. This will help keep your skin hydrated. Twenty minutes is the magic number because that's typically how long it takes to get home from a workout.

Just make sure that whatever routine you have, you like it and it fits into your schedule. Keep baby wipes or a cleanser in your gym bag, and have fun!

FUNCTIONAL MEDICINE

Functional Medicine is a newer term that is becoming common in the medical world. This practice teaches the body to function in a way that is natural and to prevent 'Dis-Ease.' If you see a functional medicine doctor, this is how they refer to the body being unbalanced, meaning we want to live with "ease" and if we put bad foods in our bodies, we live with "Dis-Ease" as we age. Functional medicine doctors practice early prevention of chronic diseases by restoring the functionality and health to the greatest extent. *Functional medicine is an evidence-based clinical approach that addresses the environmental influences and imbalances with the idea that when balanced, the body can return to its natural state of health and balance.*[34]

Functional medicine tests for allergens, metals or toxins in the body and identifies and explains any imbalances in the organs. When testing is complete, the doctor recommends supplements, dietary guidelines and individual support to stay on track and ensure the health is improving. I don't mind getting older. I just don't want to be sick, in pain or on 40 different medications when I'm 80. That is not how I envision my future life. Naturopathic and functional medicine helps. It is becoming more popular and is in high demand.

Functional Medicine Has Been Guided by Six Core Principles:[35]

1. *An understanding of the biochemical individuality of each human being, based on the concepts of genetic and environmental uniqueness.*
2. *Awareness of the evidence that supports a patient-centered rather than a disease-centered approach to treatment.*
3. *Search for a dynamic balance among the internal and external factors in a patient's body, mind and spirit.*
4. *Familiarity with the web-like interconnections of internal physiological factors.*
5. *Identification of health as a positive vitality – not merely the absence of disease emphasizing those factors that encourage the enhancement of a vigorous physiology.*
6. *Promotion of organ reserve as the means to enhance the health span, not just the life span, of each patient.*

Samantha's Story Time

Interesting story. I have a client who came in with acne because her functional medicine doctor was helping her cleanse from all the metals in her body. As she followed the program, her skin changed from clear and glowing to purging with cheeks full of acne. This doesn't happen to everyone. She just happened to have high levels of metals in her body and through the cleanse, she was purging toxins through the skin. Just because the skin is an organ doesn't mean that you will always breakout. Not everyone experiences a negative impact, and some have clear and glowing skin throughout the entire detox. For instance, I detoxed right after the holidays, even with all that sugar, I didn't have a single breakout.

If you are ready to be healthy, and work hard, functional medicine is a wonderful lifestyle choice. I have met several functional medicine doctors. I love their philosophy and how they can heal their patients with food.

Part 3: The Deep Skinny on Ingredients & Products

Samantha's Passion

Throughout this book, a great emphasis is placed on the importance of quality products that work for your skin. Everyone's time, skin and needs are different. An at-home routine can be a couple of steps or many steps. The most critical element is to find the right products for your personal skin type and conditions, then determine a consistent skin care routine to follow day and night to give your skin the best opportunity to cleanse, protect, refresh and restore.

I am extremely passionate about helping people understand the products they are using on their skin. It is one of the reasons I have become an author. When it comes to over-the-counter (OTC) products, marketing hype and celebrity endorsements are the expected and accepted norm. Often, consumers literally buy products specifically because a celebrity they like uses it. It's a tried and true formula for marketing.

I have always been curious about the amount of the markup, wondering how much the products cost to make and how much money is spent in advertising. Cosmetic chemist, author and mastermind behind BeautyBrains.com says, *"Some skincare products you can buy in mainstream beauty stores cost about two dollars to make, but retail at $300. Other skin-care products cost 50 cents to make and are sold for two dollars. And although the actual percentages of the markups is a trade* *secret that companies don't reveal, in general, these products are not using ingredients so expensive they would warrant the cost."*[36]

I've also wondered about the manufacturing process and ingredients used to make over-the-counter products and the impact they have on our overall skin and health. OTC products tend to use more fillers and harmful ingredients to make the product look, feel and smell good. Unfortunately, to market and sell the product, it needs to look good. Even though it may look good, it does not mean the product is high quality. Why is that? Because most consumers do not have any idea what the ingredient label means and how to even decipher the ingredient contents. Stacy Malkan, author and co-founder of the Campaign for Safe Cosmetics, says, *"When you pay a lot for cosmetics, you're paying a lot for dangerous chemicals such as phthalates and DMDM Hydanatoin that have been linked with cancer, asthma, allergies and fertility issues. The average woman uses about 12 beauty products every day, exposing herself to over 160 different chemicals."*[36]

Chapter 6:
Product Types

OVER-THE-COUNTER PRODUCTS – THE MANUFACTURING PROCESS

It isn't a surprise that over-the-counter (OTC) products are made in large batches to meet massive product demands. *Continental Manufacturing Chemist (CMC) has a dedicated blending room which was recently renovated in 2011; ten stainless steel blending tanks; maximum capacity of 1,000 gallons. CMC has five stainless steel filling lines. Highly flexible and customizable to fit any container. Handle viscosities up to 100,000 cps with fill sizes ranging from 0.3 oz to 275 gallon totes.*[37]

It is surprising that the formulas require so many preservatives to extend the shelf life. Products can sit in a warehouse for up to two years before they land on a shelf, in stores or in the bag at a party. Unfortunately, a long shelf life means more preservatives and fewer or no active ingredients. If the product was to include active ingredients, it would spoil too soon or lose its effectiveness.

As previously mentioned, labels may tout that the product contains vitamin C or E, which is a good thing. However, the placement of the ingredient on the list indicates whether the ingredient is a preservative or stabilizer. When the vitamin is at the top of the ingredient list, it provides a greater benefit. If the vitamin is towards the bottom of the list, it contains less than 1% of that vitamin. The last items on a product label are preservatives or stabilizers.

In stores, consumers expect to purchase multiple products for various issues. Oftentimes, it is the same manufacturer with specific lines made for skin conditions such as acne, anti-aging, rosacea, pigmentation or dark spots. At some point in our all of our lives, over-the-counter products have been a big part of our life.

Samantha's Story Time

A client of mine recently shared with me her step into 'womanhood.' She shared, "I remember when I was 14. I felt so grown up. My mom took me shopping for three things. We went to the salon to get my eyebrows shaped and waxed. We went to the department store beauty counter to get my own skin care regime which consisted of a cleanser, toner, moisturizer and a free gift in a pretty little makeup bag. Lastly, we went to a third store to have a makeup lesson done. It was one of my favorite days."

PHYSICIAN PRODUCTS

Dermatologists are necessary and helpful for extreme skin care issues. They help by writing prescriptions for certain ingredients to treat specific skin conditions. The ingredients in the products are higher amounts than OTCs, spas and professional grade products. The level of these actives allows medicine to penetrate the dermis. While OTC lines aren't supposed to penetrate through the skin's barrier (even though they strip it) and professional lines aren't meant to go beyond the Dermal/ Epidermal Junction, physician lines can penetrate to the dermis.

Sometimes this is necessary for extreme skin issues. Other times, for issues such as acne, rosacea, melasma and others, this isn't always good. If product gets to the dermis, it means the epidermis is stressed and has been compromised so it will allow the products to penetrate.

When a doctor prescribes retinol, the side effects are redness, irritation, peeling, dryness and flaking skin. Their direction is that it's normal and will subside once our skin gets "used to the product." Unfortunately, that is false. The product is irritating the skin and creating surface inflammation to trick us into thinking that our skin is less wrinkled. I should say that vitamin A is great for treating wrinkles, but not at high percentages. Anytime the skin goes into fight or flight mode, there is a wound to the skin and once the product has stopped, the skin looks worse than it did when you started that ingredient.

PROFESSIONAL PRODUCTS
Professional products are NOT all created equal. There are some lines that are not as active or beneficial as others. However, the majority of professional lines are highly active and are designed to treat the skin instead of sit on the skin's surface. The difference between professional products that are 100% active and ones that aren't is that inactive products are sold in certain stores.

Professional Grade Products – The Manufacturing Process
Live actives help heal skin conditions and maintain healthy and vibrant skin. Professional products are made in smaller batches, have a shorter shelf life and need to be used within six months. Professional lines use higher quality ingredients and focus on delivering results to their consumers and their estheticians.

I personally won't use or sell a product that I know won't deliver results. It also needs testing to prove the efficacy of the ingredients. Fortunately for estheticians, Dr. Johnson personally does his own testing and shares his published scientific data with us. He also uses estheticians as his test subjects for certain trials and we get to hear their personal experience as the trials are underway. Dr. Johnson says, *"Professional lines analyze ingredients and their purpose. For professional lines, our focus is the result."*[38]

I'm not making a case of bad versus good. We all have our preferences. I merely want to bring awareness, so you can make informed decisions on what is best for your health and skin. When we know better, we do better. Since the professional product manufacturing process requires products to be made to order, they need to be ordered, which may require a little planning. However, there are many benefits to professional grade products.

Benefits to Professional Grade Products

- Less preservatives, fillers, irritating and harmful ingredients.
- The physician or cosmetic chemist designing the product line uses a variety of active ingredients in the serums only. When active ingredients are used in a cleanser, exfoliant or moisturizer, they do not provide benefits below the surface.
- Products will not compromise the skin's barrier.
- Professional cleansers and exfoliants won't strip the skin of oil.
- Moisturizers will be thick enough to offer proper hydration levels without clogging your pores. Many professional products, even the oil-based ones, are non-comedogenic (non-clogging).
- Instead of buying several products for different skin conditions, professional products can be customized to meet the specific needs. For instance, acne skin isn't always oily and may need more moisture to keep the skin functioning properly and the barrier intact.

There are enough options out there for everyone. It's sometimes hard to make the decision, so when in doubt, seek the advice of a trusted, licensed professional esthetician who has passion for her career, a varied level of experience and significant knowledge of the products she recommends.

Looking to your esthetician for skin care products is one of the best things you can do for your skin because they understand skin, can get to know your skin and understand how your skin functions. They can also decide which products will work best and offer you the correct daily treatment protocol. Daily care and SPF coverage are the best anti-aging treatments that you can do for your skin to look younger and slow down the aging process.

As skin types change and seasons change, it is easy for your esthetician to customize the products you need. Without guessing what you need, your esthetician makes it seamless from season to season, so you can remain looking and feeling good, but most of all confident that you are taking great care of your skin and your health.

Samantha's Story Time

On a personal note, I have been using professional skin care products on my skin for the last 13 years. I can honestly say that at the age of 37 most people still believe that I'm in my late 20's or early 30's. It is because of the amazing changes I've seen in my skin and how it really has helped slow down the aging process. I am also very diligent about my routine and make it a point to never go to bed without washing my face (no matter how late or how many glasses of wine I've had). I always stick to my routine and rarely skimp on my treatments.

Over the past 13 years as an esthetician, I have used several different professional lines. The one I'm currently using in my spa has truly been amazing for both my clients and me. For me, I was able to reduce my acne and flare ups and completely cleared my skin of the Post Inflammatory Hyperpigmentation (PIH) which are those ugly red marks left behind after the acne is gone.

CHIRAL PRODUCTS

It is with deep gratitude that I dedicate this section to Dr. Ben Johnson,[38] president, founder and formulator of Osmosis Skin Care. Dr. Johnson has been a great resource, mentor, and inspiration to me as an esthetician and to me as a person.

"Chirally Correct" products are terms that scientists, chemists, physicians and estheticians use to create product. This is the method of preparation for medications, topicals and professional skin care products. Chiral products only contain the left side of the molecule that offers the ability to give desired results. Professional and physician-strength skin care products are made chirally correct, which produces results-based products that can be used at home.

Discovered by Louis Pasteur in 1847, who, after earning a doctorate in both chemistry and physics, *undertook a crystallographic study of Tartaric Acid only to find that the crystals and salts were chiral due to hemihedrism i.e. the presence of small (right-leaning) facets at alternate corners. He found this salt to be a mixture of two chiral crystal forms with right- or left- leaning hemihedral facets and related as object and its mirror image.*[39] This means that when a chemist is dealing with atoms, they can use either the right or left side in skin care formulations or medications. It is key to knowing if it is the left or right side because these ingredients need to join together in a formulation. How will they react with the other molecules in the body?

This concept can be confusing to explain to consumers who don't understand the science behind the skin. To help me with this chapter, I was fortunate to interview Dr. Johnson who explained this process in great detail. I also found a chiral article in "Dermascope," an esthetician's trade magazine.

Chirality is often described as the "handedness" of molecules. To illustrate, think of your left and right hand. They are mirror images of each other, but could you fit your left hand inside a right-handed glove? The same holds true for chiral isomers, which do not link perfectly with one another and are not superimposable but are, rather, mirror images of each other.[40] Pasteur's discovery has helped many pharmaceutical companies develop medications that are effective by using the correct side.

The Importance of Chirally Correct Products
Johnson explains, "our body is a left-handed working environment."[38]

When a product is formulated, it needs to use the left side for it to be more effective.

Samantha's Story Time

"Now, that I've used your products for a while I can see such a difference. When I first started coming to you, my face looked like raw meat. It was awful. I had been using the popular home party product, and it nearly destroyed me. I had never had a rosacea flare up like that. Your facials and products calmed it down, but even after a few months, it wasn't quite clearing up for good. The flare ups kept returning. I finally had to see my dermatologist who gave me my prescriptions. I used it for 2 weeks, the flare ups cleared up. However, I didn't want to be stay on medication, so I switched back to your line, and my face has never looked so good! I needed the prescriptions to get me out of the woods, but I didn't have to stay on them. I didn't wear makeup all summer, and my rosacea has never been so calm."

Ingredients are labeled with an 'L' or a 'D' to identify if it is formulated for the left or right. Using vitamin C as the example, on a label it is written as L- or D-ascorbic acid. L- means left and D- means right. Ascorbic acid is tricky because our skin will only absorb the L-ascorbic acid form and the D- might not provide our skin any benefit. It is also possible that D-ascorbic acid may also be used as preservative ingredients.

Generally, OTC products are not chirally correct. Therefore, the body must adjust to accept the ingredients. Dr. Johnson also shares, *"Manufacturers buy either L- or D- forms of the ingredient. L- can be less irritating and more effective on the skin."*[38] Skin is smart! It knows what it likes and will accept or it will reject any ingredient. Johnson states, *"our bodies can shift to make balance of ingredients."*[38] As we have mentioned before, the skin is an amazing organ that we have for a very long time. Like the rest of our body, we need to treat it well. Chirally correct products certainly offer that extra special, loving care the skin needs to stay healthy and natural.

Samantha's Cleanse

Our skin DOES remember all the damage, trauma, sun burns and irritation that we caused it, and it leads to accelerated aging. We need to be aware of the products we are putting on our skin. Finding the right esthetician is so important. You will want to find one that:

- can treat the skin properly from within,
- uses products that penetrate to the DEJ,
- offers the results without irritation,
- slows down the aging process, and
- recommends or carries proper actives and custom skin care products.

The last thing I'm going to say about all products, is that if you use a product and your skin either goes back to the way it looked before or looks worse than it did before you started, that product is damaging and aging your skin. Avoid any of these products and use something that your trusted esthetician tells you to use. One of the concerns I hear from clients is they are afraid of the cost. OTC and home-party products are not exactly cheap, especially when your skin does have a negative reaction. While professional products may or may not cost a bit more, because they are custom, they are more likely to work naturally with your skin. When clients spend time and money on 2 or 3 rounds of products in 3 months, they could have easily purchased professional products one time for that same 3 months. When the seasons change and the skin changes, that custom product can be adjusted, thereby giving more use for the same purchase. Finding the right product that meets your goals without pain, chemicals and flare-ups is the goal.

Chapter 7:
Know Your Ingredients

The market is flooded with skin care products. Many products can damage the skin or have harmful ingredients that accelerate aging, create sensitized skin, or increase toxins, resulting in health problems. This chapter is a culmination of several weeks of research to gain insight on how to recognize the impact of various ingredients on the skin.

PRODUCT LABELS

Reading product labels is more than confusing. Oftentimes, manufacturers use several names for the same ingredient. It's hard to believe that companies are purposely changing the name to camouflage the real products. With beauty products, a manufacturer can add less than 1% of an active ingredient and claim that it has XYZ ingredient in the product to reduce wrinkles or clear up the skin. When the amount is 1% or less, it is usually used as a preservative or stabilizer. This means the complete ingredient isn't even used as we expect.

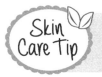

Empower yourself with how to read a label and the order of the ingredient list so you can decipher harmful versus helpful ingredients.

Alternative Ingredient Forms

When a manufacturer creates a product, they want it to sell. For marketing purposes, they add catchy words to the label to attract attention. They also know the average person will read and buy it without ever reading the ingredients list. For purposes of consistency and familiarity, vitamin C will be used as the example throughout this chapter.

Vitamin C is an ingredient that is often touted on products, but very little is used within the product. Vitamin C is an unstable ingredient. It will oxidize if it is not used either as an alternative form or is encapsulated to keep the ingredient intact. It must remain stable until it is delivered into the skin. Even then, vitamin C is a tricky ingredient because it is very unstable and will oxidize if placed in a bottle that is exposed to light or air.

There are many different forms of the ingredients that are included in a product and work better with the skin than others. As mentioned, an L- or D- may be found before the ingredient name. That letter indicates the type of ingredient used. For example, vitamin C can be seen as L-ascorbic acid or vitamin E as D-tocopherol.

When you look at the label on the back, you will never see the word 'vitamin C' on the label. You will see the words 'ascorbic acid.' Ascorbic acid alone is rarely used on a label unless it has a stabilizer ingredient to keep the vitamin C from oxidizing. However, 'Vitamin C' will be on the front label of the bottle to entice you to buy, but the exact wording is never in the actual ingredient list. There are various forms of vitamin C that are effective when used on the skin, such as magnesium ascorbyl phosphate, L-ascorbic acid, ascorbyl glucosamine and ascorbic acid. Magnesium ascorbyl phosphate is non-irritating and more stable than the ascorbic acid version of vitamin C. It is also less irritating for sensitive skins.

HOW LABELS ARE DESIGNED

Labels are put on products for our safety. When reading a product label, ingredients are listed from the largest amount of ingredients to the smallest. Manufacturers will trick consumers by stating there is an active ingredient in a serum, but when you look at the ingredient list, the ingredient is at the bottom of the label.

It is important that we are aware of certain ingredients and know what should or shouldn't be added to a product and why or why not. The problem is when a tiny amount of an ingredient is added to the product, we don't know the exact coverage or the effect it will have on us. If the ingredient is on the label, they can state on the front of the container "contains vitamin C for anti-aging" even though that is a false claim.

The Skinny on Labels

1 Water, **2** C12-15 Alkyl Benzoate, Butylene Glycol, Glycerine, Dimethicone, Glyceryl Stearate, Cetearyl Alcohol, **3** PEG 100, Stearate-2, Tocopheryl Acetate, Bisabolol, Allantoin, Laureth-7, Disodium EDTA, Propylene Glycol, Fragrance, **4** BHT, Sodium Hydroxide, Citric Acid, Phenoxyethanol, Xanthan Gum

1 Water is usually the very first ingredient and makes up the majority of the product.

2 Then the next 4-5 ingredients make up the bulk of the product, about 10-15%.

3 The rest of the list of ingredients are those that contain less than 1% of the ingredient in the product. In an OTC serum, the L-ascorbic acid is usually listed in this section, indicating the product contains less than 1% of vitamin C.

4 The last 2-5 ingredients are the preservatives.

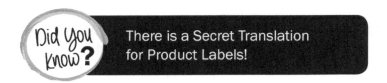

Did You know?

There is a Secret Translation for Product Labels!

Water

If you look at most product labels, water is the first ingredient and makes up about 70-80% of the product. This explains why preservatives are so important. Water adds hydration to the product and helps it stay moist. Water also adds moisture when applied to the skin.

Main Ingredients

The next 4-5 ingredients in the formula are the main ingredients that make the product feel the way it does. There is always an emulsifier, which helps to bind the water-in-oil or oil-in-water ingredients so they don't separate when sitting on the shelf.

Also, hyaluronic acid, active ingredients, encapsulation formulations and hydrating ingredients are the main ingredients in this next section. These ingredients are formulated so the skin accepts the products and it feels good when applied to the skin.

Active Ingredients

These ingredients are only beneficial when added to a serum. Many manufacturers add actives to cleansers and moisturizers. However, adding it to the cleanser is not necessary because you immediately remove the cleanser and waste the actives. As for moisturizers, the point is to sit on the skin to hold moisture. Active ingredients do not help treat the skin when they sit on the skin's surface. Actives need to penetrate.

This is where "claims" of anti-aging come into play. If an active ingredient sits on the skin's surface, it can irritate the skin. If it is causing skin irritation, the skin becomes inflamed, thus the claim of "anti-aging" because the skin swells and hides the wrinkles.

Another problem with OTC manufacturers adding active ingredients is that they don't encapsulate them. Since the products are manufactured in bulk, the products cannot be encapsulated. Encapsulated products have active ingredients which expire over a shorter amount of time. However, manufacturing smaller batches allows professional and physician product lines to include active ingredients in their products. This is very important when working with actives because most of them are very unstable ingredients and encapsulating them keeps them stable. Serums with actives need to penetrate into the Dermal/Epidermal Junction (DEJ) where the live cells are born. This is the only place where actives can actually help and treat the skin at its source. Once this encapsulated bubble gets to the DEJ, the bubble releases the active ingredients to treat the new cells. This is very important because unless the actives get to this layer of the skin, they don't help treat the skin. Therefore, it defeats the purpose to include active ingredients in cleansers and moisturizers.

Fillers as Ingredients

The use of fillers as ingredients differentiates OTC products from professional and physician product lines. Fillers are literally added to fill in space and make the product feel great on the skin. These ingredients can be used in various ways such as fillers, fragrances, or preservatives. This is where manufacturers want us to believe the product will produce certain benefits and treat the skin. However, oftentimes, they do not offer any benefit to the skin; they can be harmful or even irritating in the wrong skin types.

Fillers are mostly added in less than 1% increments of each ingredient, but if you add several fillers to a product, it adds up. They can add less than 1% of any ingredient, active or vitamin, yet claim that the product has XYZ vitamin or active added. If you look at the label, you will see the ingredient listed, but that doesn't mean that it has enough to make a difference. Also, the manufacturer can list these ingredients in any order. Once they hit the less than 1% amount and when they state that vitamin C (for example) is in this particular product, they may place it as ingredient number seven on the list.

I recently learned that some vitamins, such as vitamin E, can be used as a preservative and not as an active ingredient. Like vitamin C, vitamin E has different names and some forms are used as preservatives. However, a manufacturer may state on the front label that vitamin E has been added. A consumer without an understanding of product labels would purchase the product believing the product contains vitamin E for anti-aging or healthy skin care. Unfortunately, the consumer is not getting the benefits they think from the vitamin E because its function is to preserve the product and not to treat the skin. There isn't enough of the ingredient used to benefit the skin.

Essential oils and extracts are used in the same way. However, these ingredients are added to help make the product smell better because raw products without scents smell horrible. Be aware that most OTC oils and extracts are synthetic because they are less expensive and this does not have to be labeled, nor does the manufacturer have to reveal the source. Consumers may believe it contains essential oil, but it is a synthetic fragrance with the "essential oil name." If you were to purchase the actual essential oil, you would know how expensive it is because it takes a lot to break down certain flowers to extract the oil. Synthetic forms are listed within the category of a fragrance, but with a different, hidden name.

Preservatives

Preservatives get a bad rap, especially from the days of parabens (learn more later in this chapter) and the false studies that have been in the media for several years. We do need preservatives in the products for our safety and to prevent the growth of mold, fungi and bacteria in cosmetics. For their extended shelf life, OTC products must contain higher amounts of preservatives than professional or physician product lines. The higher amount of preservative helps ingredients hold up to the elements and to last on the shelf before its purchased and opened. Even after the product is purchased, preservatives protect the formula from the heat, moisture, light, air and dirty fingers.

Some preservatives are now hardly used in products, such as DMDM hydanatoin, methylisothiazolinone, some of the ureas and/or triclosan. These ingredients have formaldehyde-releasing properties. The more commonly used preservatives are phenoxyethanol, citric acid, vitamin E (tocopherols), benzoic acid and xanthan gum.

As you can see there is a lot to decipher in product labels. Hopefully, this chapter provides good information for you to understand how to read the labels and how to be more aware of the ingredients used on your skin.

THE DIRTY THIRTEEN OF BEAUTY PRODUCT INGREDIENTS

This chapter is not about food. It is about skin care product ingredients that have the potential to harm our skin and our bodies. In order to identify correct information and misinformation, I researched data from and interviewed cosmetic chemists, product manufacturers, and fellow estheticians. This chapter is offered to provide you with an awareness of ingredients, how they are used in beauty products and why certain ingredients are used. As with any product, be mindful and avoid using certain ingredients in every beauty product you own. However, keep in mind that some do have their benefits for certain formulations, like shampoo and conditioners.

It was eye-opening to perform extensive research and get to the bottom of the claims that we read or hear about in the news. It was also enlightening to find out whether the information is true or false with proof from scientists and chemists. This list is both proof and my opinion. As you shop for products, keep it with you to read product labels to help you determine what ingredients work for both you and your family. Always keep in mind any allergies or sensitivities to prevent negative reactions.

I've mentioned my good fortune to discuss this topic with Dr. Johnson who helped shed light and offer suggestions. Dr. Johnson shared,

"Estheticians choose healthy and effective ingredients and look for what makes physiological sense."[38] Estheticians are in the treatment rooms educating clients on products and ingredients. The question that helps him gain perspective is, *"Are they doing harm to change the skin?"* He encourages us to *"think independently to see if results are permanent and create real change in the skin."*[38]

Sodium Lauryl Sulfate/Sulfite

Sodium lauryl sulfate or sulfite (SLS) in its natural state is used to degrease engines and is the main ingredient in garage floor cleaners. Sodium lauryl sulfate/sulfite is found in products like shampoo, facial cleansers, toothpaste, hand soaps, baby soaps or shampoos and shaving creams. Cosmetic chemists put SLS in these products because this is what gives the cleanser its foaming ability. In excess, SLS may damage the skin's immune system or potentially cause young eyes to become underdeveloped.

In 2003, a German study was done to test the difference in skin reactions between three detergents; sodium lauryl sulfate (SLS), sodium laureth sulfate (SLES) and alkyl polyglucoside (APG). Different concentrations of each ingredient were tested with various exposure times and the skin was tested for Transepidermal Water Loss (TEWL). *We found a pronounced reaction to SLS, and a far milder one to SLES. Even at the highest concentration, the skin reaction to APG was hard to detect.*[41] The skin was tested again at days 3, 7, and 10 and by day 7, SLES was no longer detected as irritating, but SLS was still showing irritation after the 10-day mark. *These results demonstrate the improvement in reduction of skin irritation achieved by development of novel detergents.*[41]

Alternative detergents can be used in cosmetics:[42]

- Saponins are natural cleansing agents found in some desert climate plants.
- Decyl Glucoside, a mild, nonionic cleanser is used for sensitive skins. Although you will not see this ingredient listed alone, it works best when combined with the following ingredient.

- Cocamidopropyl Betaine is derived from coconut oil and gentle on sensitive skins. If you are allergic or sensitive to coconuts, avoid this product (please note, this is derived from coconut oil; it is not the actual coconut oil itself which can clog the pores).

Propylene Glycol

Propylene glycol acts as a surfactant or wetting agent in products in its natural state. It is the main ingredient in anti-freeze, de-icing solutions for airplanes and can clean barnacles from boats. Factory workers are required by the FDA to wear protective clothing when producing products that contain propylene glycol and are required to dispose of them as toxic waste. We read things like this and immediately think that this ingredient is bad, but there are different grades of propylene glycol. The grade used in antifreeze is not used in beauty products.

Propylene glycol is an organic alcohol, which stabilizes formulas and dissolves natural extracts in products. *In the U.S., it is listed as GRAS (Generally Recognized as Safe) for use in food and pharmaceuticals in the U.S. Food and Drug Administration document.*[42] However, propylene glycol in high concentrations can cause skin irritation and has a drying effect on the skin. It has the potential to dissolve the intercellular cement in the skin, which causes Transepidermal Water Loss (TEWL). Alternatives to propylene glycol include butylene glycol or glycerin which show better tolerance in the skin and very minimal skin irritation or TEWL.

Diethanolamine (DEA), Monoethanolamine (MEA) or Triethanolamine (TEA)

These ingredients are known as hormone-disrupting chemicals that can cause cancer-causing nitrates. In 2010, the Cosmetic Ingredient Review Expert Panel opened up the 1983 safety assessment of all three ingredients. If you are a science-geek like me, the index has a link to all three studies. If not, here is a brief overview of all three.

Diethanolamine

(DEA) in its pure state is a white solid at room temperature. It is water-soluble and acts as a coolant, which makes it act like a liquid. It is used to prevent corrosion. DEA is used in cosmetics and shampoos as a pH adjuster, surfactant, emulsifying agent, hair or skin conditioning agent, foam booster and antistatic agent. In cosmetics, DEA is used to give the product a creamy texture and foaming action. DEA is used because it can absorb water and most products are mostly made of water.

DEA is a potential skin irritant to exposed workers and has been tested on mice. However, these tests expose the mice to the pure form, start low and increase until they see a reaction. Humans and mice don't react in the same manner! *The CIR Expert Panel concluded that DEA, an ingredient that functions in cosmetics as a pH adjuster, is safe for use in cosmetic formulations designed for discontinuous, brief use followed by thorough rinsing from the surface of the skin. Because of the potential for irritation, the concentration should not exceed 5% in products intended for prolonged contact with the skin.*[43] DEA can also be toxic to aquatic animals if exposure becomes too high.

When used in products, very small amounts are added and trace amounts may be seen. On labels, you will see DEA as cocamide DEA, DEA-cetyl phosphate, DEA oleth-3 phosphate, lauramide DEA, myristamide DEA, and oleamide DEA.

Monoethanolamine (MEA)
MEA is also known as ethanolamine, a colorless liquid that smells similar to ammonia and is part of the lipids. MEA is used to remove gases, such as carbon dioxide, by keeping the acid-base of the gases controlled.

MEA is used as a buffering agent or in preparation of emulsions, which is a water-in-oil or oil-in-water solution that stabilizes the product to maintain its texture and prevent the product from separating. You will see MEA listed on ingredient labels as MEA and MEA-sulfite in cosmetics. MEA-Benzoate and MEA-Salicylate are used as preservatives. *This ingredient was reviewed by the Cosmetic Ingredient Review Expert Panel, and concluded MEA-Salicylate is safe as used when formulated to avoid skin irritation and when formulated to avoid increasing the skin's sun sensitivity, or when increased sun sensitivity would be expected; directions for use include the daily use of sun protection.*[44]

Triethanolamine (TEA)

TEA is a clear liquid but can solidify in cool temperatures. TEA neutralizes fatty acids and solubilizes oils that are not water-soluble, which means that it is used as an emulsifier. It can be a mild skin and eye irritant but only in formulations over 5%. When a formulator adds TEA to the product, less than 1% is used. T EA *has been reviewed by the Cosmetics Ingredients Review Expert Panel that concluded that TEA and related TEA-containing ingredients named in this report are safe as used when formulating to be nonirritating.*[45]

TEA functions as a surfactant, skin conditioning or hair conditioning agent, and pH adjuster to cosmetics. TEA is used in many leave-in conditioners for hair products. Some common names for TEA products include, TEA, TEA-lactate, TEA-lauryl sulfate and TEA stearate. TEA-sorbate functions as a preservative for products.

Polyethylene Glycol (PEG)

Polyethylene glycol can be used in cosmetics as cleansing agents, solubilizing agents, emulsifiers, skin conditioners, emollients or solvents and this all depends on the type of PEG used. There are hundreds of variations of PEG, but the most commonly seen ingredients on a label include PEG-number.

When testing these PEGs, scientists and chemists used undiluted formulations on mice and guinea pigs in various percentages and tested until a reaction occurred. They also used concentrated patches on humans and left them on the skin for various amounts of time. When I read this, I recognized that they are literally looking for a reaction and test in high doses until a reaction occurs. The problem is that the high amounts of these ingredients would never be added to a product. When chemists add PEGs to an ingredient, the usage ranges from 5% to -1%. Skin irritations can occur, but in concentrations less than 1%, it is unlikely that PEGs are the skin irritant.

Many PEGs do not penetrate through the skin's barrier and are used as a filler or "fluffy" ingredient to make the product feel good on the skin. Some PEGs are occlusive, meaning they can trap the pores from oxygen and when the pore can't "breathe," blackheads can form.

Sodium Hydroxide

Sodium hydroxide is salt-based, also known as lye. Sodium hydroxide is used in soap and is water-soluble, which is why it is used in cosmetics and is used by one company in the production of aluminum. Sodium hydroxide can digest tissues and was used by serial killers to turn dead bodies into soap. If it touches the skin, it will instantly burn. Sodium hydroxide is used in food preparation to wash or chemically peel fruits and vegetables; olives soak in a sodium hydroxide solution to turn them black and preserve them in the can.

For safety, the Cosmetic Ingredient Review Expert Panel reviewed this ingredient in 2014 and published the data in 2015. *The CIR Expert Panel concluded that Sodium Hydroxide and other Inorganic Hydroxides such as, Calcium Hydroxide, Magnesium Hydroxide and Potassium Hydroxide are safe in hair straighteners and depilatories under conditions of recommended use; users should minimize skin contact. These ingredients are safe for all other present practices of use and concentration described in this safety assessment when formulating to be nonirritating.*[46]

Sodium hydroxide is used to balance the pH of products and mainly develop bar soaps, but can be used in cleansers, shampoo, body lotions and some baby products.

Triclosan

Triclosan was recently banned in soaps and cleansers because it is known to damage the skin. Its chemical structure is similar to that of Agent Orange. Triclosan was added to antibacterial products to reduce or prevent bacterial contamination. I mentioned earlier in the chapter that the main ingredient in almost all products is water, which can breed mold. The FDA currently is investigating and researching triclosan for its safety and effectiveness. In the meantime, avoid use until studies proving its safety or danger are published. According to the CIR Expert Panel, *Triclosan may bind to estrogen and/or androgen receptors and thus may act as an endocrine disruptor.*[47]

Triclosan is used in toothpaste, mouthwash, antibacterial soaps or sanitizers, hand, body and face washes, deodorant, shaving cream and wipes along with household cleaners, which means exposure can come from either inhalation or contact via the skin. Triclosan is found in our water in wastewater plants and there is no way of removing it, which causes harm to our animals and aquatic life.

Most reviews have suggested that triclosan is slowly and not extensively absorbed by the dermal route, consistent with its low water solubility, but is rapidly and well absorbed by the oral route. In human subjects, for example, daily use of triclosan-containing toothpaste for up to 65 weeks resulted in increased blood levels compared to pre-use levels, but those increased levels remained steady and returned to baseline after use.[47] This info has been published in 2010 when the CIR Expert Panel reviewed triclosan. The FDA is requiring extensive testing because it needs to ensure the safety for the consumer. I rarely see Triclosan on an ingredient label, but you still need to read labels because it is inexpensive to use and manufacturers may occasionally slip it in.

DMDM Hydanatoin and Urea

DMDM hydanatoin and urea are ingredients known as formaldehyde-releasers. They are used as preservatives to prevent the growth of bacteria, mold and microorganisms in our cosmetics and are there to ensure our safety during use of that particular product. OTC products have higher amounts of preservatives to keep them from expiring for 3-5 years; professional products have lower amounts and expire within six months to one year.

When formaldehyde-releasers come in contact with water, they generate formaldehyde. Some water-soluble formulations can cause a chemical reaction, which depends on the pH level of the formula, temperature of the solution and the length of time the product is stored. There are many preservative products that do not release formaldehyde and work well to preserve our products.

The ideal preservative should have the following properties:[42]
- *A broad spectrum antimicrobial effect at low concentrations and optimal pH*
- *Combination of bactericidal and fungicidal effects*
- *Low allergenicity and toxicity, and be nonirritating*
- *Stability and water soluble*
- *Compatibility with other ingredients (i.e. be both colorless and odorless)*
- *Ease of use*

The FDA considers urea (by itself) to be GRAS (Generally Recognized as Safe) when used in concentrations between 1-10%. Urea is used as an exfoliant to help dissolve the intercellular glue which holds the skin cells on the surface; this would allow certain products to penetrate the skin. Urea is also used in OTC cream depilatories, moisturizers, hair conditioners and teeth whiteners.

Diazolidinyl Urea is a preservative and is considered safe in cosmetics in concentrations up to 0.5%. *The Cosmetic Ingredient Review Expert Panel recognized data gaps regarding use and concentration of this ingredient.*[48] More research needs to be done. Until then, avoid use of this ingredient.

DMDM Hydanatoin is a formaldehyde releaser and works as a preservative because of its ability to keep the product from developing microorganisms. There is not a lot of new information about DMDM Hydanatoin, and it is most likely in the process of review and testing for safety. Hopefully, more information will come out soon regarding this ingredient.

Parabens

Parabens have such mixed reviews and with all the misinformation out there, it's difficult to know what is true and what is false. Parabens have been used in beauty products as a preservative because they provide a broad-spectrum protection against microorganisms. We do need preservatives to prevent the growth of microorganisms. When used in beauty products, parabens are non-irritating and non-sensitizing but can cause skin irritation to those who are allergic.

According to the American Cancer Society, although parabens have weak estrogen-like properties, the estrogens that are made in the body are hundreds to thousands of times stronger. So, natural estrogens (or those taken as hormone replacement) are much more likely to play a role in breast cancer development.[49]

The paraben study that was done stated parabens were present in breast tissue of breast cancer patients. Unfortunately, there were no non-cancer patients studied and the information, therefore, is inconclusive. According to Dr. Johnson, *"Parabens are able to form a tumor or have the ability to encapsulate themselves in a tumor." Parabens are used less often in beauty products; this ultimately led to the demand for paraben-free products. I recommend that parabens should be avoided and kept out of our products, especially if studies, even though proven inconclusive, show that they have the ability to form in a tumor."*[38]

Another concern is what are manufacturer's replacing parabens with? Several of the newer preservatives are formaldehyde-releasing ingredients. Just because parabens have been removed, doesn't mean that our products are any better for our skin. When reading a label, you will see parabens listed as methylparaben, propylparaben, butylparaben or benzylparaben. Methylparaben is the most effective and commonly used.

Alcohol, Isopropyl or SD-40

SD in any alcohol preparation means that the alcohol has been denatured, or "Specially Denatured" (SD). These are used in cosmetics and a variety of products. Alcohol in higher percentages can be drying or irritating to the skin and may strip the skin of its moisture barrier, which creates microscopic holes in the skin's surface. In addition, bacteria can enter and skin sensitivity increases. *Denatured Alcohols, in the U.S., must conform to the Code of Federal Regulations (CFR) specifications for completely and specifically denatured alcohol.*[50] SD alcohols are added to cosmetics to function as an antifoaming agent, astringent or solvent.

The difference between isopropyl alcohols and SD alcohols is that isopropyl alcohol mixes with either water or alcohol. It is insoluble in salt solutions and can be separated by adding salts. This causes the isopropyl alcohol to separate. Isopropyl alcohol is used in hand soaps, disinfecting solutions and hand sanitizers. We are all familiar with rubbing alcohol; this is isopropyl alcohol and quickly cleans the skin. Isopropyl alcohol can depress the central nervous system and we can get headaches, dizzy, nausea, vomiting, hypothermia or shock from excessive exposure. I use isopropyl alcohol in my spa to keep my wax pot and work surfaces clean. I get a headache if I do a lot of cleaning or my room is closed up.

SD alcohols are composed from ethanol, which have to be denatured to become a solvent. There are hundreds of denaturing methods and additives that could be added to the alcohol. This is why there is potential for skin irritation or sensitivities. We do not always know the additive ingredients.

Mineral Oil

Mineral oil is a derivative of petroleum and goes through a refining process to be used in cosmetics. It is used in oil-based products as an emollient for dry skin types and protects against moisture-loss in the skin. Mineral oil can create a film or barrier on the skin that traps ingredients in the skin, almost like applying plastic wrap. This film can prevent the skin from properly shedding. Mineral oil is highly comedogenic, and it will clog your pores. The film created by mineral oil can also interfere with the skin's ability to eliminate toxins, promote acne or other skin disorders.

FD&C Color Pigments

ALL cosmetic colors have undergone extensive testing and are not allowed unless the FD&C approves the color. Colors are tested in batches. The FD&C must approve each batch before a manufacturer is allowed to use that color in any ingredient for food, cosmetics or medications.

When you see FD&C before a color, it means the Federal Food, Drug and Cosmetic Act (FD&C) has approved the color under their strict system for color additives. Certified colors have three things added when reading a label: prefix, i.e. FD&C; color name i.e. Yellow; and Number, i.e. No. 5 (FD&C Yellow No. 5).

Colors can be labeled another way, called 'Lake' which are not water-soluble, but are used to prevent bleeding in lipsticks. *A lake is a straight color extended on a substratum by absorption, coprecipitation or chemical combination that does not include any combination of ingredients made by a simple mixing process.*[51]

If your product (except coal-tar dyes) contains a color additive, by law you must adhere to requirements for:[51]

- *Approval – all color additives used in cosmetics (or any other FDA-regulated product) must be approved by the FDA. There must be a regulation specifically addressing a substance's use as a color additive, specifications, and restrictions.*
- *Certification – in addition to approval, a number of color additives must be batch certified by the FDA if they are to be used in cosmetics (or any other FDA-regulated product) marketed in the US.*
- *Identity and Specifications – all color additives must meet the requirements for identity and specifications stated in the Code of Federal Regulations (CFR).*
- *Use and Restrictions – color additives may be used only for the intended uses stated in the regulations that pertain to them. The*

regulations also specify other restrictions for certain colors, such as the maximum permissible concentration in the finished product.

The only color that has not undergone testing are colors from plant, animal or mineral sources, which are not subject to batch testing like FD&C or Lake color pigments. They are color extracts and natural sources, which can cause skin irritation because some people may be sensitive or allergic to certain plants.

If you would like to check the colors yourself, reference number 52 is a link to the U.S. Government Publishing Office's Electronic Code of Federal Regulations, Part 74 – Listing of Color Additives Subject to Certification.[52]

Fragrance

As explained in Part 2, there are 4,000 ingredients that make up fragrances. Many are not regulated and can possibly be carcinogenic. Fragrances that are harmful can cause headaches, dizziness, allergic reactions, skin discoloration, violent coughing, vomiting and skin irritations. Fragrances affect the nervous system and can cause depression, hyperactivity, irritability, behavioral changes and the inability to cope. Fragrances are a topic of controversy because the FDA does not regulate fragrances even though it can cause skin sensitivity. Manufacturers can add phthalates into products via the term "fragrance." I'm hoping that over the next several years, fragrances will be included in strict regulations for labeling.

When consumers learned about the sensitivities and lack of regulation, they started seeking "fragrance-free" products. The problem was, the ingredients that are used to create the product do not smell nice and fragrances are added to make the product appealing for both sales and for use. Who wants to use stinky shampoo or body wash? Therefore, fragrance-free products have some fragrance in them to mask the real scents of the original materials.

Ingredients in a product are required to be added to the label.

However, manufacturers can put an unregulated ingredient on a label as a "fragrance," even though it is not approved by the FDA. *In most cases, each ingredient must be listed individually. But under U.S. regulations, fragrance and flavor ingredients can be listed simply as "fragrance" or "flavor."*[53] The FDA does not have the same power to regulate ingredients in cosmetics as it does with our food. Unfortunately, certain ingredients fall between the cracks and get put on a label or renamed to hide that ingredient. This, too, can result in skin irritations, sensitivities and allergic reactions.

Fragrance and flavor formulas are complex mixtures of many different natural and synthetic chemical ingredients, and they are the kinds of cosmetic components that are most likely to be "trade secrets."[53] Essential oils aren't always the answer because many people are allergic to certain plants or the extracts they produce. Be cautious when purchasing beauty products. When in doubt ask your esthetician to recommend a product that is less irritating and has the right fragrance.

There are many fragrances that will not cause harm and are safe for use on the body. Professional products gravitate towards these fragrances because they need their products to smell good as well.

Phthalates

Phthalates (pronounced Thay-lates) are a group of chemicals that are used in hundreds of products, such as toys, vinyl flooring and wall covering, detergents, lubricating oils, food packaging, pharmaceuticals, blood bags and tubing; and personal care products, such as nail polish, hair spray, aftershave lotions, soaps, shampoo, perfumes and other fragrance preparations.[54] Some of the more commonly used phthalates are dibutylphthalate (DBP), dimethylphthalate (DMP) and diethylphthalate (DEP). DBP and DMP are rarely used, but DEP is still widely used in cosmetics.

Phthalates also get into our body by food consumption. Phthalates are used in the production of plastic. *Though most foods indicate low or no*

detectable residues of phthalate esters, fatty foods show higher residues.[55]
This means that phthalates are getting into certain foods, and we are ingesting them when we eat. Dairy products seem to show higher levels of phthalates getting into the food from the plastics used.

Phthalates have been used in cosmetics for many years and are still undergoing testing for toxicity and skin irritation. *All phthalates considered here have a low dermal toxicity in the range of 3-20 g/kg, which is well above the expected use levels in cosmetics and [bug] repellents. However, the long-term effects of such exposure are unknown.*[55]
Phthalates in cosmetics can either be sprayed into the air via hair sprays or put into the water via cleansers, soaps or shampoos.

No matter the use, they harm the environment during production, use or disposal. The proof is minimal, but the study done by the EPA does state that: *in every study where DBP was tested, it is reported as the most toxic phthalate. DBP's effects, as well as those of other phthalates, were generally observed at levels greater than 1mg/1.*[55] This is especially harmful for aquatic animals because fish can rapidly absorb toxins and harmful ingredients versus humans and other aquatic mammals.

If we eat fish that has high phthalate levels, we will increase the potential for toxicity in our bodies. Shrimp, crab and other seafood that are lower in the food chain tend to have the highest amounts of phthalates. Salmon had inconclusive results for having both high and low levels of phthalates. However, salmon tend to be more susceptible to absorbing certain pollutants than most other fish. *The U.S. EPA has stated that acute and chronic toxicity to freshwater aquatic life occurs at concentrations as low as 940 ug/l and 3 ug, respectively, and may occur at lower levels for more sensitive species (U.S. EPA 1980). Based on a review of the data available, concentrations of phthalates affective aquatic organisms were usually greater than 1000 ug/l, ranging in 1900 ug/l to over 10,000 ug/l (section 5.2).*[55]

Phthalates are also found in water and in the plastics used to bottle our water. To avoid this exposure, buy bottled as little as possible and only use BPA-free reusable water bottles to fill throughout the day. There is inconclusive data that shows phthalates can cause cancer. *Recent data on carcinogenicity and the estimations of exposure suggest that criteria, standards, or other regulations in relation to phthalate esters, specifically DEHP, may need to be re-examined.*[55]

Many of these ingredients use less than 1% in most formulations, but when you are using 20+ beauty products on a daily basis, that number increases and your exposure levels to these ingredients also increase. I did find one piece of information interesting: *The Federal Food, Drug and Cosmetic Act (FD&C) does not authorize the FDA to approve cosmetic ingredients, with the exception of color additives that are not coal-tar hair dyes. In general, cosmetic manufacturers may use any ingredient they choose, except for a few ingredients that are prohibited by regulation.*[56]

SUMMARY

This chapter isn't meant to scare you. It was designed to offer you the truth and testing behind each ingredient. For further information, see my list of trusted sources in the reference section in the back of the book. Keep in mind that there are multiple sources online offering poor information. It took me over two weeks to write this particular chapter because I wanted to make sure that what is written here is proven and multiple sources confirm the information.

If you would like to conduct your own research, I highly recommend doing so. Also, keep these sources handy because new ingredients will always come under fire. You do not need to believe every story in the media. There are chemists and scientists who do believe in the safety of the consumer, and their job is to study ingredients until proven safe or unsafe.

Chapter 8:
Makeup

TYPES OF MAKEUP

Various types of makeup are used daily by both women and men. However, makeup is probably the most misunderstood product on the market. There are thousands of brands, products and ingredients that can either be helpful or harmful to the skin. It can clog, dry and irritate. Ingredients that are harmful, such as lead, can be used in the manufacturing process. Educating yourself to make informed decisions will support skin care goals.

COSMETICS

Women choose makeup to improve their appearance and boost their self-esteem because when a woman looks good, she feels good. Whether makeup is used daily, weekly or for special occasions, those who use it are familiar with the different types of products and their uses.

1) **Foundations** are typically powder or liquid. Newer formulas go on like powder but offer full-coverage like a liquid. Full coverage foundations hide uneven skin tone, redness or breakouts. New on the market are BB and CC creams which are applied like a facial moisturizer. These formulas provide full coverage as they treat the skin, but some may feel heavy.

2) **Blushes and/or Bronzers** are designed to highlight the cheeks and give a pop of color, especially in the winter months when skin tends to look dull and pale.

3) **Concealers** hide dark circles, blemishes, redness and uneven skin tone. Concealers can contour the skin to enhance the best features.

4) **Eye shadows** come in a wide variety of colors and formulations. Colors help draw attention to the eyes to match outfits and transform the eyes from day to night.

5) **Eyeliners** are available in gel, pencil or liquid form to line the outer edges of the eye. Depending on the look desired, the pencil is used for daytime, and gel or liquid is used for a bolder look at night.

6) **Mascara** comes in curling, lengthening, volume or waterproof formulas. Mascara draws attention to the eyes by lengthening the eyelashes.

7) **Eyebrow pencils** are becoming popular as women want a full, filled-in brow. They are available in pencil, gel or a mascara-like formulation to add color to your brows. Those new to eyebrow pencils can start with the gel or the pencil and apply lightly. It is always easier to add than remove eyebrow makeup. Brow mascara wands keep the eyebrow's shape while adding a touch of color.

8) **Lip pencils** are used in gel or pencil form to help lipstick last longer throughout the day. Lip pencils work best when lips are hydrated. Before using the pencil, apply a light layer of lip balm to help it glide on easier.

9) **Lipsticks or Lip Glosses** are used to give lips color. Colors range from light, pale pinks and nudes to bright reds, purples and oranges to enhance the lips and transform your look from day to night. I love to use light pinks during the day and add red or fuschia when I meet friends for drinks.

MINERAL MAKEUP

Even though camouflage makeup must be of the mineral variety, not all mineral makeup is created equal! Over-the-counter (OTC) companies offer both non-mineral and mineral-based foundations in either liquid or powder forms. Be careful when choosing mineral makeup because OTC lines use ingredients that can irritate the skin.

Certain ingredients used in mineral makeup can give the skin a reflective look, causing the skin to look shiny or washed-out in photos. Certain minerals used in makeup are not beneficial to the skin. There has been controversy around titanium dioxide powders stating they can cause harm when ingested. However, titanium dioxide is important for the SPF protection.

Commonly used mineral makeup ingredients are:

- Titanium dioxide protects the skin with SPF.
- Mica offers a healthy glow to the skin, but can look reflective in pictures. It is not always recommended for foundations, but works great in eye shadows.
- Bismuth oxychloride has natural antiseptic properties and can look reflective in pictures. Bismuth oxychloride, if not ground down properly, can embed microscopic particles into the skin and potentially cause skin irritation. For sensitive skin or acne, do not use a foundation containing bismuth oxychloride.
- Iron oxides are pure pigments that leave the skin looking smooth and natural.

Mineral-based eye shadows are very effective, because they use iron oxides to make the colors bold and visible. Unfortunately, iron oxides do not last as long as regular shadows.

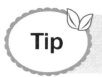

Tip
For mineral eyeshadows to last longer into the day, dab a light layer of concealer on the eyelid as a base.

There are countless options for selecting the right makeup for ourselves. The more we learn about it, the better the choice for our skin.

STAGE MAKEUP

When working in theater, it is important to apply enough makeup because the stage lights affect the actors' appearances. Stage makeup or theatrical makeup is heavy and has bold colors to stand up to the bright lights onstage. Stage makeup can enhance or change the person's look with a different application. Once light is added to the stage, various types and colors of makeup can accentuate the character's features. Here are some examples:

- Pink lights can intensify warm colors or dull/gray cool colors.
- Bright red lights are not recommended because they can disappear. For example, light to medium reds fade, and dark reds turn brown.
- Yellow lights turn orange and cooler shades gray, or even black.
- Amber or orange lights intensify makeup. For example, reds turn orange or cool colors turn gray.
- Green lights can gray all tones and adding yellow and blue intensifies green.
- Blue lights can gray most tones or cause them to look red or purple.
- Purple or violet lights can darken oranges or red, and blues can look more purple.

Since the camera is further away from the actor, the makeup needs to be more dramatic and use more colors. The pigments in the makeup use more dyes, so foundations tend to be heavier. The heavier the product used, the higher risk of clogging the pores. Many actors have skin problems because they wear heavy stage makeup for several hours each day.

Estheticians or makeup artists who apply stage makeup tend to be specialized in this area. They take specific makeup courses to understand how the light affects the skin. Most theater makeup artists specialize in stage makeup and have an extensive portfolio to showcase their talent.

HALLOWEEN MAKEUP

Halloween is a fun time of year when we get to put on gory, fake, crazy makeup to make ourselves look scary or silly. Halloween makeup can be very toxic or irritating to the skin because it's inexpensive, thick and contains heavy dyes. Consumers don't want to spend a lot of time applying Halloween makeup before heading out. I highly recommend doing a patch test on your forearm to make sure that the makeup won't irritate your skin.

10 Tips for Purchasing Halloween Makeup:

1) Buy makeup made from natural pigments to avoid artificial colors and skin irritants.
2) Make sure the makeup kit says non-toxic!
3) Avoid harmful ingredients such as emollient laxatives, talc, hydrocarbons, or kohl.
4) Be aware that Halloween makeup can cause lead poisoning!!! Avoid anything that lists kohl, kajal, al-kahl, or surma.
5) Halloween makeup must be approved by the FDA.
6) Glow-in-the-dark makeup should be avoided because there is little research done on the safety of the colors.
7) Do a patch test prior to applying on the face and around the eyes.
8) Follow all directions carefully. If a product says avoid eyes, it will irritate them and cause possible damage!
9) Protect your skin! Apply a primer before applying Halloween makeup. This minimizes clogged pores. Without a primer, any possible skin irritation may worsen. The primer may also help give a smooth finish.
10) Don't forget to wash it off! Don't go to bed with your Halloween makeup on because this makeup WILL clog your pores and cause breakouts.

The FDA has a list on their website that shows the safer options when purchasing cosmetics. *Additional information on color additives can be obtained from the Color Additive Status list on the FDA website.*[57]

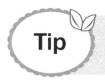

Tip When in doubt, avoid using Halloween makeup unless you want to risk skin irritation or clogged pores just to look funny or scary on Halloween.

Camouflage Makeup

Camouflage beauty makeup is an amazing gift that estheticians and makeup artists use to help camouflage scarring, post-accident trauma, post-surgery or during cancer treatments. It is such an honor to help re-instill the confidence of beauty sometimes lost in these situations.

First of all, the makeup line needs to offer top quality ingredients that will not clog or irritate the skin. The skin needs to remain healthy as it heals. Camouflage makeup artists or estheticians take additional training courses to learn:

1) specific techniques to hide the scarring or hair loss; and
2) how to teach their clients to properly apply their makeup at home.

Professional camouflage product lines are lightweight and designed to keep the pores clear. Camouflage makeup is used as a foundation or can be applied to the skin in a specific area prior to applying a different foundation. Many camouflage makeups are waterproof for the day to prevent rubbing off if the skin weeps or sweats after an intense workout. Color matching is very important, especially when the makeup is applied under the foundation. The key is to not bring attention to darker or lighter areas, but instead appear seamless with a natural appearance.

When I was in oncology esthetics training, we learned about camouflage makeup so we can help our clients with:

1) applying a lightweight foundation on their skin during chemo or radiation treatments;
2) drawing eyebrows; and
3) making eyelash marks look natural.

These quick and easy tips make our clients look and feel confident. Oncology-approved makeup is available to estheticians. It must use non-irritating ingredients without any dyes. It also must be mineral-based without ingredients like bismuth oxychloride or talc, so it does not irritate their already delicate skin.

MAKEUP INGREDIENTS

Makeup has evolved since the days of lead-based makeup or the kohl that the ancient Egyptians wore. They had many great inventions with skin care, but their makeup was toxic and caused a lot of damage to their skin and eyes. Even with makeup, there are good and bad ingredients. Comedogenic ingredients clog the skin and cause blackheads, so it is important to be able to decipher the ingredient list before buying.

Controversial SPF Protection

Titanium Dioxide is used for SPF protection and has been the subject of great controversy as a recognized, possible carcinogen. The state of California went under fire with concerns about titanium dioxide. Fifty thousand titanium dioxide products were tested for safety and found the suspected toxicity concern was unfounded. In July of 2015, California voted in favor of Proposition 65. *The Safe Drinking Water and Toxic Enforcement Act of 1986 was enacted as a ballot initiative in November 1986. Proposition 65 requires the state to maintain and update a list of chemicals known to the state to cause cancer or reproductive toxicity.*[58]

Best Makeup Ingredients

With all the makeup lines on the market, there are plenty to choose from. While some contain harmful or irritating ingredients, there are others that compliment a healthy skin care regimen. Many professional lines are light on the skin, while still providing desired coverage. Most professional makeup lines (sold exclusively in spas and salons) are like skin care products. While offering the same attractive look, they will contain fewer ingredients, fillers, dyes, and lower preservatives.

Harmful Makeup Ingredients

The FDA does not require companies to test all ingredients used in cosmetics for safety. This means that bad ones can slip in because they keep the manufacturing costs down. Makeup should never leave the face shiny or give your skin an unnatural glow. Some products have the potential to get into our bloodstream and harm our skin and bodies. The following list provides several ingredients to use with caution and several have been further explained earlier in Chapter 7.

1) **Phtalates** (they-lates) are endocrine disruptors that also go by the names of dibutylphthalate (DBP) or diethylphthalate (DEP).

2) **Lead and Heavy Metals** Lead is a proven neurotoxin. Mercury is harmful to various systems in our bodies, it also harms the environment and wildlife. These metals may be listed as lead acetate, chromium, thimerosal, hydrogenated cottonseed oil and sodium hexametaphosphate. *Note: Lead is no longer used in makeup, but years ago, eye pencils, shadows and lipsticks were all lead-based. Ancient Egyptians used lead-based makeup daily, and they were left with scarred skin, health problems and even suffered from mental health conditions due to lead poisoning.*

3) **BHA and BHT** are known endocrine disruptors and can also harm wildlife and the environment.

4) **Formaldehyde Releasers** are potential carcinogens. Some common names are DMDM, hydantoin, diazolidinyl urea, imidazolidinyl urea, methenamine and quarternium-15. *Note: Quarternium, also known as quats, are used in hospitals, spas and salons to disinfect and keep tools safe from bacteria and spread of disease. These are the only approved materials for disinfection. In my spa, I use great caution when cleaning and disinfecting my brushes, wands and other tools that come in contact with my client's skin. We are still getting exposed to these chemicals on a daily basis in the hospital, medical, salon or spa environment. The safety of our clients is most important and quats are proven to be effective.*

5) **Carbon Black** is a potential carcinogen for the lungs and cardiovascular system.

6) **Talc** in its natural state, contains asbestos. Talc used in beauty products has been asbestos-free since the 1970's. Asbestos-free talc could potentially cause ovarian cancer in women and is no longer recommended for use in cosmetics. Many non-mineral foundation powders also contained talc but many manufacturers no longer use it.

7) **Kohl** was a paste made from soot or fatty matter and metal, such as lead, manganese or copper. It caused eye irritations, irritability, insomnia and mental health problems. Kohl was the main ingredient in eyeliners and mascara. Up until the mid-1960's, it was still widely used in the makeup our mothers, grandmothers and great-grandmothers wore.

8) **Rat poison** was used many years ago to formulate eyebrow or eyelash dyes and even early eyelash growing formulas. Rat poison is no longer used, but could have affected our grandmothers and great-grandmothers.

Read labels on all cosmetics. When in doubt, try another line or consider professional lines from your esthetician.

MAKEUP'S REVENGE

Samantha's Cleanse

When I walk around a department store, I see every makeup counter with rows upon rows of foundations, beautiful eye shadows, lipsticks, glosses, mascaras, eyeliners, brow pencils and gels. Isn't it fun to sample the selections? Most of the counters offer disposable Q-tips, foundation wedges and lip or mascara wands for sampling. That's clean, isn't it? How many of us have used them? Or do we actually use our finger in the foundation or eye shadow to test it on our hand? Then, do you touch the next one and repeat until you find that perfect shade?

Let me ask you a question... When you are hanging with friends at the appetizer counter, do you double-dip in the dip bowl? Then WHY on earth would you double dip from the makeup palettes at a department store? You do not know where other people's fingers have been. Maybe you use the wedges or have clean hands, but others may not.

When I think about the amount of bacteria in the sample makeup selections, it grosses me out. It makes me cringe at the thought of having my makeup done for an event. Those color palettes harbor so much bacteria from dirty fingers and brushes touching them, it's amazing more people aren't suffering from conjunctivitis or eye infections.

Let's talk dirty. It doesn't matter if the makeup is a sample or it is your own. All of it contains bacteria at some point, if not cared for properly. Bacteria leads to skin irritations, breakouts, and eye infections.

Tips to Clean It Up

This section is going to focus on the bacteria that can be harbored in makeup palettes and why they need to be cleaned or no longer displayed in stores. I am going to discuss the importance of keeping your makeup brushes clean and how to properly clean them, because dirty brushes can lead to skin irritation, acne or eye infections (even when using your own products). I'm going to talk about why you should toss makeup that's older than one year and how much harm you are doing to your skin and eyes by keeping the old stuff.

Scenario - Makeup Palettes

It is a luxury to have someone else apply our makeup, and it is a fun event, especially when with friends. Department store makeup artists absolutely keep their brushes clean. However, the problem lies in the transfer from the dab of the brush to the makeup palette, to your cheek and back to the palette. The dirt, oil and dead skin cells from your cheek just left an imprint in the palette. This imprint, call it DNA if you like, is now waiting for the next clean brush to pick it up.

Problem

This is a problem, especially if you suffer from acne. Double dipping will transfer the bacteria back into the foundation palette which eventually will be applied to someone else's skin. Not to mention all the dirty fingers that have touched it before your makeup application.

In addition, anytime the eye is involved, makeup should never be double dipped. Eyelashes have microscopic bugs, called follicle mites. Follicle mites are beneficial because they keep out infections and harmful bacteria that could potentially enter into our eyes. However, when transferred from one person to the next, they are harmful and could cause irritation or infections to others.

Solution

In esthetics school, we were given tools to squeeze or scrape the makeup we needed into a tray. We then applied that makeup to our client. We used multiple mascara wands and sterilized lip and eyeliner pencils. We scraped off lipstick from the tube and dabbed the gloss onto our palette to be applied via a disposable lip brush. Ask your makeup artist to scrape or squeeze the foundations, eye shadows, bronzers, concealers, lipsticks and glosses to keep yourself safe from bacteria.

Scenario - Clean your Makeup Brushes

We clean our bedding, pajamas and towels regularly because we know they harbor bacteria and get smelly. The same rule applies to makeup brushes, especially if you suffer from acne. Makeup contains preservatives to keep bacteria from growing during the transfer of makeup to skin or eyes. Professional makeup lines have lower preservatives than over-the-counter (OTC) makeup lines because they are made in smaller batches and are meant to be tossed after six months (just like skin care products).

Problem

If you suffer from acne, you may use concealers and foundations to cover the blemishes. Bacteria transfer from your brush to your skin and from your skin to your makeup palette. Those who suffer with continuous acne breakouts should wash makeup brushes every day. If not, acne bacteria are spreading around your face as you apply makeup and add new bacteria to the brush, palette and skin.

Solution

Whether or not you suffer from acne, keep your brushes clean.
- On a daily basis, a brush cleaner containing alcohol will work for a quick wash.
- However, be sure to wash the brushes weekly with baby soap and water with time to air dry. Wash with baby soap once a week, unless suffering from severe acne, then use daily.

Makeup artists and estheticians spray brushes after every application. We also wash them with soap, water and disinfectant to protect our clients. Our makeup brushes touch a lot of faces and we need to take every necessary precaution to keep our clients safe from bacteria in the makeup and our brushes.

Scenario - Toss old Makeup

In my 20's, I had a giant makeup bag with every eye shadow color. I loved having my eye shadow match my outfit. I loved turning my daytime look into a dramatic look for night. When I had my oldest son in 2007, I finally went through that bag. Realizing they were several years old, I tossed them out because they were filled with bacteria. Now that I am a mom of three kids, my makeup routine is super-simple and only takes five minutes. I am down to a palette of three eye shadows that I wear for work and evenings out.

Problem

Makeup has preservatives to prevent the growth of fungus, mold or bacteria that could harm our skin or eyes. These preservatives are meant to last for only so long, and once that product expires, the preservatives are no longer effective. If you keep makeup for too long, it harbors bacteria and can cause eye or skin irritation.

Solution

While it is fun to have different shadows and create different looks, it is not easy to remember how long you have had it. A good rule of thumb is to check your makeup every six months to one year. If you haven't used it in a while or you don't use it frequently, toss it out. Most makeup does not emit a sour odor to indicate it is expired, and using expired makeup is counterproductive to taking good care of our skin. When in doubt, throw it out!

CAUTION ABOUT DIY PRODUCTS

In recent years, Do-It-Yourself (DIY) recipes for facial scrubs, exfoliants, masks and makeup have been shared on social media. In an attempt to be healthier or save money, people are venturing into these trends without proper information. If you are someone who loves making your own lipstick or lip balms, good for you!

It takes a lot of time and money to create these products. Be aware of how they are applied. Know that natural foods are not necessarily chemical free. Even when a product or an ingredient is natural, it does not always mean that it is good for the skin. Sometimes putting a raw or natural ingredient on the skin can create immediate inflammation or some type of skin reaction.

Part 4:
Estheticians & Spa Services

Chapter 9:
Properly Trained Estheticians

Many years ago facials were considered a luxury spa service. That is no longer true; there are many benefits to having facials. Facials have come a long way since the 1980's when the skin was stripped and peeled to the point of extreme redness and irritation. No longer are the days where you leave the spa after the facial with a bright red face. Before a treatment, the first question many ask is, "Am I going to leave here red and irritated?" The answer is "no." In this chapter, I want to create awareness and educate about the important role an esthetician plays in your health and well-being. Facials are no longer a luxury, but rather a necessity.

> *"You should have your Esthetician on speed dial."*[60]
> - **Lori Crete**, Esthetician, Spa Owner, President
> and Founder of "The Esthetician Mentor"

ESTHETICIAN TRAINING

Estheticians go to school to receive their license in esthetics. Some estheticians are licensed cosmetologists, who also learn how to care for skin, but not to the extent of estheticians. Although, every state is different and continuing education class (CEU) requirements vary, the State of Illinois requires estheticians to complete the following to earn and keep their license:

- 750 hours of school that teaches science, biology, history and spa care
- 10 hours of CEU's every 2 years to keep the license current

THE LIFE OF AN ESTHETICIAN

Our education teaches us how to give a fluffy facial and has the same set of training to get us ready for the state boards. Once we pass our state boards, we venture out to find a job doing what we love best, facials! Sounds simple right? Wrong!

I spoke with Abbie Major, licensed esthetician and owner of Abbie Major Skin Love.[59] She says *"I was an esthetician robot who did what I was told to do. However, I did not feel passionate about skin care. I just went through the motions. I knew I was good at my job, but I just didn't believe in what I was doing."*[59] Unfortunately, many estheticians feel the same. If we do not have a respectable mentor or find an industry niche, many in the field move on to other careers. The skin care industry is saturated with spas on practically every corner, so it is difficult to find a job and build clients. The quality of care varies from spa to spa, as well as the quality of products.

My first job was in a medical spa. I soon realized that was not my niche. After three years, I moved to a day spa in town. The owner took me under her wing and taught me everything: how to give a proper facial, how to study the skin by reading and feeling it as I service the client, and how to treat each client individually. Major's mentor is Dr. Johnson. Major read his book, Transform Your Skin Naturally, and she explains, *"It resonated with me on every cell of my being. I found my new path, my passion and my calling! I never looked back. I BELIEVE in what I do now. It all makes complete sense to me. It's like an awakening. I was asleep before just going through the motions. Now, on a very deep gut level, the puzzle makes sense. Being a natural wellness esthetician makes sense to me. I feel authentic and in alignment with my purpose and passion!"*[59]

THE UTTER IMPORTANCE OF AN ESTHETICIAN

Having a mentor fueled my passion for skin care. It is important to find an esthetician who has this same passion for skin because they will serve you the facial treatments your skin needs. Many consumers have fallen into purchasing the ever-popular online daily deal for their facials and spa treatments. When someone spa hops from one deal to the next, it is very difficult to help heal the issue. Consistent treatments are best because the skin gets what it needs. Lori Crete, licensed esthetician, spa owner, president and founder of The Esthetician Mentor, says *"I would love to see the extreme discounting go away and instead, have clients search for high quality care and professionalism."*[60]

Why should you have your esthetician on speed dial? As Crete mentions, *"professional, high quality and consistent treatments comprise the most effective approach to skin care and spa services."*[60] The care that professionals offer does make a significant difference in meeting your skin care goals for a healthy look. You'll even feel better, too.

During the 60-minute treatment session, we are physically touching your skin to properly 'read' it and know what it needs. Furthermore, we can provide professional grade products that are custom to your skin's needs. You can't get that type of assessment in a fifteen-minute doctor appointment. Dermatologists are highly trained doctors and can help those who have severe skin issues. Less severe concerns like acne, rosacea, uneven skin tones or melasma can and should be treated by an esthetician.

Skin problems all stem from inside, and we lead you to heal the skin from the inside and the outside. Crete believes the number one reason why consumers should seek out the advice of trusted esthetician is, *"to receive result-based solutions from an educated professional."*[60] Obviously, you are interested in a healthy lifestyle since you are reading this book. I am grateful for your purchase. Thank you. The treatments my spa provides are natural healing-based solutions, which are determined by the needs of your particular skin during your facial. Healing from within lasts longer and has so many benefits to overall health. If health is your goal, teaming up with a trusted, experienced, passionate esthetician is the right thing to do.

Chapter 10:
Spa Services

REALITY CHECK

Beauty is influenced by the media and celebrities never seem to age. Even well into their 40's and 50's, they appear flawless. There are never indications of wrinkles or cellulite and their skin looks like satin. With a little airbrushing in our photos, we would look flawless too. And then people would see us in person. That would be scary. We have become conscious about wrinkles and aging because of the media. What they show is not real. It's impossible because even my 3-year-old has little lines around her mouth when she smiles.

Celebrities are paid for their looks. I do not begrudge them. They work very hard at the gym with personal trainers to stay in shape and they have cooks who prepare healthy, low-calorie meals. While the rest of us Americans enjoy our food, celebrities are under tight scrutiny to consistently watch their diets.

In addition, celebrities have teams of stylists, hair, makeup and estheticians to make them look gorgeous. Celebrities use high-end professional products and see their esthetician regularly for facials and add-on treatments because they need clear skin. The makeup applied for the camera is heavy, thick and clogs their pores. Surprise. It's hard to believe, but under the heavy makeup, many celebrities have acne, especially when filming.

Most people are not celebrities. However, we can maintain care to look and feel our best. Face lifts and injections are not necessary because there are many alternative treatments to highlight the youthful beauty in each of us.

It all starts with YOU! Are you willing to change your perspective and think about your skin and your lifestyle? What steps are you willing to change to get monthly facials and use the correct home care with professional products that will give your skin exactly what it needs? Let's examine the options.

ALTERNATIVE SKIN CARE

My first recommendation, if you don't already have one, is to find an esthetician who is knowledgeable, passionate and educated. You want to make sure the esthetician keeps up with continuing education and is engaged with their business.

You deserve to have the best for your skin. This may require you to switch from current products that may not be working for you. In time, when you are ready, the professional grade products can bring benefits that will enhance the feel and look of your skin. These spa grade products have active ingredients, but do not contain fillers or irritating ingredients that will harm your skin or cause inflammation to 'hide your wrinkles.'

Once you find your esthetician, do everything she tells you. She knows. During your first facial, your esthetician is getting to know your skin and can feel what's going on by touch and how your skin responds to the products that are applied. We use this knowledge to design your skin care program. Always ask your esthetician for add-on treatments that can boost the effectiveness of your facial.

Add-on services may include:
- Microcurrent
- Oxygen facials

- LED light therapy
- Peels or Non-Acid Peels
- Microdermabrasion
- Ultrasonic facials
- Microneedling (depending on the state)

When there is a desire to treat skin conditions or to establish a healthy glow and clear complexion, an esthetician will definitely help you reach those goals. The purpose of this book is to educate you as best we can, so you can make informed decisions about your skin care. As you take the next step to talk with estheticians, cosmetic representatives, and independent representatives, you will know the questions to ask that will help you best find the right solutions for you. Estheticians love when clients are knowledgeable about their skin because it helps open the lines of communication to determine the best plan for treatment. In addition, we can make the necessary shifts as needed to ensure your skin feels its absolute best.

AN ESTHETICIAN'S MACHINE LIST - TOOLS FOR ESTHETICIANS

When it comes to finding the right esthetician, it can be overwhelming. Each spa has its own tools, products, services and machines. The quality of care is not based on the number of machines in a spa. It is not "the one with the most machines wins." Some estheticians work with one machine and focus on that specific service or niche.

I operated my spa for five years before purchasing my first machine. After extensive research, I decided upon the microcurrent machine. It made sense for me because I want to keep up with the needs of my clients. Microcurrent services are non-invasive and give immediate results. There are several machines and product lines to choose from.

Most Common Facial Treatment Machines (aka modalities)

These types of machines are optional modalities for estheticians to offer various services to their clients. In this chapter, we explain how these are used and the benefits of the service.

- Ultrasonic
- LED lights
- Microcurrent
- Laser
- IPL (Intensed Pulsed Light)
- Microdermabrasion
- High Frequency
- Microneedling
- Radio Frequency
- Oxygen Machine

When your philosophy of skin care matches with the esthetician and her/his belief about the reasons for certain machines and services, it is a perfect match!

EXFOLIATING

To Exfoliate or NOT to Exfoliate

Exfoliation is a topic that is starting to hit home with many people because there are so many harsh exfoliants on the market, and we are over-exfoliating our skin. Each time we exfoliate, whether it is an OTC scrub, microbeads, at-home rollers or chemical peels, the skin's barrier function is compromised. This creates more damage and skin sensitivities by stripping and over-stripping the skin.

Types of Exfoliants

The following types of exfoliants can be purchased over the counter, in spas, in department stores and from independent representatives. Following this list, we explain each one and give you as much information as you need to make informed decisions about which service may work best for you.

- Facial scrubs
- Enzymes
- Chemical peels
- Microdermabrasion
- Mechanical Scrubbing Brushes
- At-home rollers

Product Facial Scrubs

There are tons of facial scrubs on the market, ranging from apricot kernels to super-gentle microbeads. There are several types of scrubs that are included in the cleanser, for use on your face after cleansing, or to mix with your facial cleanser.

Manual Facial Scrubbers

Manual facial scrubbers work similarly to a scrub, but use a brush to exfoliate the skin. Brushes come with soft or rough bristles. Some may be sold with a scrub to exfoliate even more.

Impact to the Skin

- Manual scrubbing can be very drying and can strip the skin.
- Rubbing beads, no matter how gentle, can damage the skin's barrier by creating microtears. Microtears create little holes in the skin's barrier, which can allow moisture to evaporate off the skin's surface, increasing risk of dehydration. The tears can also create pathways for toxins and irritating products to enter the skin and the bloodstream.
- When we feel a tight "squeaky clean" on the face, it means the skin has been stripped of oil.
- When Transepidermal Water Loss (TEWL) occurs from scrubbing, the skin will become dehydrated because the skin's barrier is not fully intact.
- Manual facial scrubbers remove more dead skin layers than a scrub product, which will increase the dryness.
- Brushes need to be cleaned and sanitized between uses because they can spread bacteria.
- Acne sufferers should not use them because they can create more breakouts and transfer bacteria around your face.
- Lack of moisture in the skin leads to dryness.

Chemical Peels

Chemical peels remove unnecessary skin cells and compromise the skin's barrier. Is this a good thing? No. Why? It compromises the skin's barrier. Peels actually do more than create microtears. They remove too many layers of dead skin cells in the stratum corneum depending on the depth of the peel. This creates surface inflammation, and the skin swells to protect itself from harm.

Peels can be performed by a licensed esthetician in either a spa or medical setting. Depending on the type of chemical, most are done with Alpha Hydroxy Acids (AHAs) that work at lower pH levels to remove a few layers of the stratum corneum. Peels can consist of lactic acid, glycolic acid, mandelic acid or malic acid (all AHAs), salicylic acid (Beta Hydroxy Acid, BHA), phenolic or TCA peels. Most are done in a spa setting but some TCA and phenolic acid peels are performed by a physician because they have a lower pH and are used for resurfacing the skin.

After the peel, the skin looks "plump" and less wrinkled. This is because it is inflamed and irritated from the harsh chemicals. These are not good for the skin because the organ enters into fight or flight mode to fix the barrier and prevent further damage. Because the skin is busy healing, it may forget about current conditions, such as rosacea, acne, dark spots or melasma. Any time a wound to the skin is created, the skin has to forget about the current condition and work to repair the new wound to keep the barrier intact.

At-Home Rollers

Samantha's Cleanse

CRINGE!!! Recently, the market started selling 'at-home rollers' which are hand-held metal rollers with spikes which are rolled on the face to 'make' the product penetrate the skin. It is meant to mimic the treatment called microneedling. Microneedling is a service that is performed by a licensed esthetician, physician, nurse or nurse practitioner. The state of Illinois does not allow licensed estheticians to provide this service. Microneedling is considered a cosmetic service and must be performed by a physician or nurse. This begs the question as to why these products are allowed on the market.

At-home rollers can damage the skin more than scrubs that cause microtears, which are extremely serious. Another concern is that they are being sold by salespeople who are not properly trained in skin. A scrub would be better to use than the rollers because estheticians may not be able to repair damage from the rollers. However, scrubs are still not the solution. If at-home rollers are used, see an esthetician to determine the extent of the damage.

Enzymes

In Chapter 3, we learned that enzymes are a healthy, natural alternative to scrubs. They are applied to our skin in a gentle massaging manner, and it feels very good. All cells contain protein. As the skin cells die off, the protein remains. Enzymes work to eat (yes, enzymes are technically called a proteolytic which means they eat protein) the proteins in our skin cells that should have been removed. As you remove the enzyme, the cells come off, leaving the skin's barrier intact. Your skin is rehydrated as it utilizes the ingredients from the enzymes.

Enzymes only need to be used 1-2 times a week and are very effective at removing dead skin cell build-up. If you have sensitive or dry skin, an enzyme will work well to help hydrate the skin. Acne clients benefit from an enzyme two times a week because it minimizes clogged pores and rehydrates the skin from harsh acne products.

Microbeads

Microbeads are little plastic beads that have been added to creams as a form of exfoliation and range in size up to 1mm. Microbeads have recently been banned because *they are made from synthetic polymers, such as polyethylene, polylactic acid, polypropylene, polystyrene or polyethylene terephthalate.*[61] Microbeads are designed to be rinsed down the drains, and unfortunately, these microplastics eventually enter the aquatic habitats. *It is calculated that eight trillion microbeads per day are emitted into aquatic habitats in the United States, which means that the US emits enough microbeads to cover more than 300 tennis courts daily.*[61]

The other issue is how the terms, "plastic" and "biodegradable" are defined. *In Illinois, legislation defined "plastic" as something that retains its "defined shape during a life cycle and after disposal" which allows microbeads to be made from plastics that biodegrade slightly, thus changing their shape in an unspecified period of time.*[61]

More states are banning microbeads, and manufacturers are being forced to find a new source for exfoliants. Some of the replacements include ingredients like apricot kernels (apricot scrubs have been around forever) which are extremely harsh and irritating. Many nut-based exfoliants can cause a reaction due to an allergy or can over-exfoliate the skin to create even more inflammation than the microbeads.

Living a healthy lifestyle leads to using as many natural products as possible that do not damage or irritate the skin. Enzyme-based exfoliants made with natural ingredients meet these requirements, especially because they work for all skin types and can be used once or twice a week.

Facials

Samantha's Story Time

My grandparent's house was my second home. My grandma Dotty and I would have our special time, which included an 'at-home facial.' She would sit me over one of those face steamers to "open up my pores" with a towel over my head. We applied a peel-off mask to our faces. When it was time to remove it, we stood together in front of her mirror to see who could peel it off in one piece. She won every time.

As an esthetician, there are many different types of services we can offer. When I was in esthetics school, we were taught that masks were applied to specifically adjust the skin's pH levels back to neutral. With this approach, the moisturizer would be absorbed, staying hydrated after the facial. Every facial ends with a mask, which is how we rebalance the skin and calm any irritation that might occur from extractions.

Generally, masks, whether from a spa or store, are designed for a specific skin type. Clay-based masks are designed for acne, oily skin or to clean the pores. Creamy and gel-based masks target hydration.

While in treatment, professional masks by estheticians are formulated differently than the ones you can purchase from a spa or store. In a spa setting, estheticians use multiple masks on the face depending on the issues the client is having that day. The ingredients are specifically selected, formulated and mixed to customize the mask as needed.

Today, professional products used for treatment in spas are designed to keep the skin's pH levels steady throughout the facial. However, if performing a chemical peel, the pH levels are brought to an acidic state in order to remove dead skin from the stratum corneum. During any other type of facial service, the skin is being treated for its specific needs and every client has more than one concern with her face on any given day. This is why multiple masks are always used.

If you look on social media, such as Facebook, Twitter, Instagram and Pinterest, the "newest trend in facial masks" is called #Multimasking. The funny thing about this is that estheticians have been treating clients with more than one type of mask to target multiple skin concerns for years. This is now hot on social media and is a great benefit that clients get a "behind the scenes" view of the treatments estheticians can provide.

WHY FACIALS?

Why not? Everyone experiences skin conditions at some point in their lives. Licensed, experienced and trusted estheticians offer non-invasive services which avoid antibiotics and harsh products. Today's services do not send clients home feeling red, raw and irritated. Estheticians spend a full hour examining and treating the face with you. They are passionate about skin and offer customized facial treatments and personalized home care products. In that hour, they are touching your face to understand what it needs. Skin changes over the years, and estheticians can make adjustments as needed. While using natural products and modalities that are healing, not hurtful, estheticians can help you look and feel your best at any age!

The Process of Facials

To achieve the goal of healthy skin, monthly facials are usually recommended. However, after the facial, continuing the healthy treatment is not going home to use the same old care products. The purpose of the facial is to be sure that the products you use meet the goal to look healthy. The following outlines the facial service experience for most estheticians.

- Appointment is scheduled.
- Esthetician meets the client for a consultation with questions about the client's health, diet, lifestyle, home care and family skin history.
- Review currently used products and ingredients
- Identify skin care goals
- Examine the face with the light to feel the texture, check pore size, skin damage and anything that might be under the skin.
- Proper cleansing removes dirt, oil and makeup from the skin.
- Apply enzyme with or without steam to remove build up and prepare the face for extractions.
- Perform the extractions to remove blackheads, whiteheads and any acne breakouts. The extractions are critical during active breakouts because it gives a chance to deep clean the skin.
- Add a calming serum to reduce any surface inflammation.
- Customize a serum that specifically targets the client's skin.
- Massage serum to relax client and stimulate circulation and lymph flow. Circulation helps the skin absorb the serum into the skin. The lymph flow can remove any sinus congestion as well as

any toxins or fluids that may be stored in the face. Massage also stimulates the facial muscles to tighten, which explains why the skin looks great post-facial.

- Apply customized mask and massage to increase circulation. Masks can help calm and rebalance the skin to make it look fresh. If necessary, multiple masks can be used to work on different areas.
- Protect skin with a zinc-oxide sunscreen moisturizer for hydration and protection without chemicals.
- Brush mineral powder to remove shine.
- Create a customized home care program, personally mixed and matched based on personal skin needs.
- Send client on their way feeling beautiful with healthy, glowing skin without redness or irritation.

Many of us have memories of using peel-off or pore-clearing masks that left our skin feeling tight and dry. These masks should be used minimally because the pore-clearing masks are designed for those with oily and heavy acne. Some people enjoy weekly masks and some estheticians still recommend a mask treatment every week. Personally, I feel that if my clients schedule monthly facials and use proper skin care at home, additional at-home masks are not necessary. Regular monthly visits allow estheticians to track skin issues and adjust products and services as needed.

THE MAGIC MACHINES

Estheticians have a variety of machines called "modalities" that create better results with treatments. They provide greater product penetration and can help heal skin with acne, rosacea, surface inflammation or scarring. Every esthetician has a preferred treatment plan. Whether or not an esthetician has one modality or all, the important aspect is how they use it to properly treat the condition for which the modality is designed. A good esthetician will explain each treatment and offer personalized treatments based on your specific needs.

Ultrasonic

Ultrasonic transmits ultrasound waves through a hand-held wand. This process aids in exfoliation and enhances product penetration. Ultrasonic facials are very relaxing, and they have a soft, gentle, vibrating action that can gently remove surface blackheads or oil pockets. The soft, metal blade works to gently exfoliate the skin's surface. Since ultrasound does not remove any skin layers, which causes inflammation, the skin's barrier is left intact. The vibration forces product to reach the dermal/epidermal junction where the live cells are formed.

This procedure is recommended for clients with dry, dehydrated, sensitive or rough skin. It also helps those with dead skin build-up, melasma and rosacea.

LED Light Therapy

LED light therapy is applied with either a hand-held device or a panel that is placed over the entire face. Hand-held LED devices work well to target specific areas of the face or neck. Panel LED machines can target larger areas, like the entire face and neck. Both types work for different clients' needs. I have personally worked with both hand-held and panel-type devices and witnessed impressive results with both. I found the hand-held device to be more effective for acne. It was easier to target specific inflamed areas of the face with a focus on cystic acne bumps. It also reduced swelling more quickly.

The color of the LED lights is red, green, amber or blue. Each color penetrates at a different depth and treats specific skin conditions.

Red LED light is used to
1) lighten uneven skin tone and melasma
2) promote anti-aging
3) stimulate collagen and elastin

Green LED light is used to
1) fade freckles

2) fade brown patches
   (green light isn't as strong or effective as red light and really isn't used as much)

Amber LED light is used to
1) reduce skin redness, irritation and small facial veins
2) improve lymphatic drainage
3) flush waste from the skin

Blue LED light is used to
1) treat acne and rosacea
2) calm inflammation in the skin

Laser

More commonly known for laser hair removal, laser treatments can also be used to address various skin conditions. Lasers have different penetration rates and work to target specific areas of the face and neck. Treatments are traditionally performed in the office of dermatologists or plastic surgeons, but spas now work with doctors or nurse practitioners to offer the treatments.

Many physician-strength lasers perform a resurfacing-type treatment to remove layers of skin to help even appearance, i.e., reducing acne scars. These are harsh treatments and require downtime. Downtime means that the skin can be red, inflamed and possibly worsen over the course of two weeks. No sun exposure is recommended during this time because the skin is healing and repairing itself.

The lasers are also beneficial to reduce wrinkles, stimulate collagen, and target uneven skin tone, dark spots or melasma. Lasers have come a long way over the last 15 years, and estheticians can now perform some of the less invasive-type of laser services, IPL or photo facials (depending on the state).

Intense Pulsed Light (IPL)
IPL treatments are a light therapy, which targets the hair and skin.

However, the light frequency does not deeply penetrate because it is not technically a laser. This allows estheticians to offer the service without the direction of a physician or nurse practitioner. IPL treatments also work to remove uneven skin tone, reduce wrinkles and lighten the appearance of acne scarring. They are less intense and may take longer for the skin to respond to the treatments, depending on the type and training of the technician.

Microdermabrasion

Microdermabrasion was wildly popular 13 years ago as I finished beauty school. It was offered as a substitute to dermabrasion, which could only be performed by a physician because it literally removed the entire epidermis, leaving the skin raw, inflamed and weeping (oozing) for several weeks. Dermabrasion was designed for clients with severe acne scarring as well as deep wrinkles. However, the long-lasting damage was intense because any sort of sun exposure, even through a window, could cause irreversible damage. Therefore, patients could not leave the house until the epidermis finished rebuilding. Many clients also noticed a line of demarcation along their neckline where the dermabrasion treatment ended. This mark is permanent.

However, microdermabrasion came onto the scene so spas could perform the treatment without physicians. Every spa offered it because people loved how it could remove layers of skin to reduce fine lines and wrinkles. While less harsh than dermabrasion, it can remove up to four layers of the stratum corneum (SC). Microdermabrasion uses either crystals or diamond-tipped wands to remove layers of the SC in the epidermis to create a mild resurfacing effect. Over time, it is the equivalent of a full dermabrasion treatment. The more SC layers that are removed, the more the skin has to work to repair itself and protect itself from further damage.

Microdermabrasion was successful because we all walked around with swollen skin and no wrinkles because the skin was "plumped up." Unfortunately, many people who had multiple rounds of microdermabrasion (myself included) have aged more quickly because of the damage to our skin's barrier.

As an alternate method, some estheticians now offer a layered effect which combines chemical peels and microdermabrasion to remove SC layers. This procedure causes the skin to clear up because a wound has been created and the skin is too busy repairing the barrier from damage that it forgets about the problem the client had (acne, rosacea, melasma, etc.). The end results are clear skin and less wrinkles, but the skin is constantly working overtime to repair the barrier from damage. Once treatment stops, the skin becomes more wrinkled and the skin's conditions reappear.

High Frequency

High Frequency supplies the pores with oxygen, which allows it to breathe, reducing the breakout more quickly. It is a treatment that has been used for many, many years and is still available because of its noticeable benefits. High frequency is anti-inflammatory, anti-bacterial and reduces acne inflammation.

A Bit of Acne 101

Before acne erupts on the skin, the clogged pore does not have an oxygen supply, so the body treats it as an infection. The white blood cells rush to that clogged pore and "fight" the dirt and oil trapped inside. This is why we feel the breakout before it is visible; we feel the white blood cells "fighting." The result is a nasty red bump. High frequency emits an uncomfortable little zap. However, all of my clients have a love/hate relationship with the treatment because it decreases inflammation much more quickly than other options.

Microneedling

Microneedling is controlled wounding to the skin that stimulates the increase of collagen and elastin production for the skin to repair itself. Estheticians are not allowed to offer this service in some states because tiny needles are used to create a micro-perforation in the skin that can penetrate to the dermal/epidermal junction (DEJ). This area is where live cells are born. Estheticians must receive extensive training in order to perform this service. They need to know how to control the wound before the skin begins to bleed.

The benefit of microneedling is the opportunity to increase the penetration of products through microscopic wounds. When product reaches the DEJ, it is able to treat the live cells as they are being born. This allows product to penetrate to the DEJ. If the new cells are treated, they are healthier as they rise to the skin's surface.

Unfortunately, microneedling also creates a skin wound. So again, the concern lies with the swelling and inflammation to the skin's surface. However, it does not strip the skin of moisture because it is penetrating product.

Since this is an aggressive treatment, it is highly recommended not to combine it with additional services. Prior to treatment, a client must prep his/her skin at home for a few weeks to ensure the highest level of effectiveness. In addition, post-care is extremely important as the skin goes through its repair phase. Gentle moisturizers, vitamins, essential fatty acids and sunscreen are important products to use at home as the skin heals.

Radio Frequency

Radio Frequency is not widespread in the esthetics industry. Some estheticians love it and others do not agree with how it impacts the skin. In the process, a thermal device emits radio frequency waves to temporarily displace the skin cells to increase product penetration. The purpose is to heat the dermis in order to stimulate collagen. The heating effect on the dermis requires cooling of the skin's surface to prevent burning.

The treatment is designed to reduce aging by creating a tightening effect on the skin that combats sagging, wrinkles and overall aging. Immediate benefits are noticeable, but results usually occur about 4-6 weeks after treatment. Radio frequency can be performed in a medical spa setting by a trained esthetician, nurse, nurse practitioner or physician.

Oxygen Therapy

Oxygen therapy provides the cells with oxygen, so pressure against the skin increases. Oxygen is then diffused throughout the entire epidermis, plumping the skin to reduce wrinkles and decrease inflammation. Supplying oxygen to the pores rapidly decreases acne inflammation. In addition, it calms and soothes the skin to aid in healing scars from microdermabrasion or surgery.

Oxygen treatments are controversial among estheticians because some believe that adding extra oxygen to the skin creates free radical damage. For instance, when our skin gets damaged from the environment, such as the sun or pollution, it is called Reactive Oxygen Species (ROS). During this process, the atoms in our cells lose an oxygen molecule. This makes the atom incomplete, which it then steals an oxygen molecule from another atom. The more incomplete atoms, the more they steal from another complete molecule. This vicious cycle continues and is what causes the aging process to escalate. The more ROS in our skin, the more damage that can occur.

Microcurrent

This section is dedicated to Shari Rinaldi Braund,[62] licensed esthetician and owner of Skin Caring by Shari; and Abbie Major,[59] licensed esthetician and owner of Abbie Major Skin Love. Special thanks to both Shari and Abbie for generously sharing your personal experience, professional application and microcurrent history with me. Your guidance was exactly what I needed, as information is not yet available online about this wonderful treatment for our clients.

Microcurrent offers a safe, non-invasive alternative to injections and face-lifts while keeping the skin's muscle tone in shape as we age. It is currently the most popular facial service in the industry and used by most celebrities. In fact, celebrities have been looking for alternatives to injectables and surgeries for a while. We owe our thanks to them for urging the development of a less invasive approach to anti-aging.

For several years, I had been deciding which machine would work best for my clients. I monitored the microcurrent results and reviews for a long time. I executed extensive research and observed successful results from fellow estheticians. The results were transforming for their clients, so I decided to schedule a treatment with a colleague. My skin looked and felt amazing. It was the first machine for my spa, and I am extremely happy with the results my clients are achieving to reach their optimum skin goals.

What is Microcurrent?

Microcurrent uses an electromagnetic current to work with our body's own natural energy source to lift, tighten and tone the face. It stimulates the facial muscles to rebuild and tone, as well as stimulates collagen and elastin bonds to restrengthen and help to smooth wrinkles. Microcurrent aids in product penetration and improves skin tone. I can literally erase my client's forehead wrinkles and crow's feet, tighten up their jaw and neckline and even minimize the effects of their smile lines without injectables or face lifts. It is my new favorite treatment.

Abbie Major raves about microcurrent as it is, also, her favorite tool in her treatment room. Major explains, *"Microcurrent is based on sub-sensory electromagnetic stimulation that clears energy blockages, promotes skin health, and supports muscle re-education. This teaches the lines in your face not to be lines anymore and retrains the droopy parts to not be droopy! It also brings blood flow into the skin, which heals and feeds it. My clients literally feel better and more energetic!"*[59]

Shari Braund refers to microcurrent as *"a natural modality that the body recognizes. It doesn't hurt the skin nor the body. It offers age-reversal and makes other cells younger by stimulating ATP."*[62] Electromagnetic current stimulates our facial muscles to tighten and tone. She further explains, *"Microcurrent reconstitutes the electromagnetic energy field around the cell which is important for the gates at the cell membrane."*[62] The gates in the cell membrane allow the cell wall to open and allow water or products to enter. *"When this field is weak, the pull to open and close is slow. Microcurrent helps the pumps at those gates work better."*[62] Microcurrent also stimulates the collagen and elastin bonds to re-strengthen, which means longer lasting results for wrinkles and sagging skin. Microcurrent will smooth out superficial fine lines and wrinkles.

Microcurrent technology has the ability to penetrate products by softening the lipid barrier (the glue) that holds our skin cells in place. Once this barrier is softened, product is able to reach the dermal/epidermal junction (DEJ) to hydrate, treat and repair the new cells in the basal layer of the skin.

Microcurrent Treatment Process

Microcurrent machines have multiple settings and modes depending on the type of treatment. Depending on the machine, different light modalities, frequency, time and intensity of the signals can be adjusted to meet the client's personal needs. The different light frequencies target specific muscle depth and can remove blockages in the skin so the microcurrent can target the muscles.

My clients love taking before and after pictures because they can see immediate results and notice the results lasting longer after each treatment. Most clients need 6-8 weekly treatments to achieve the full result. Some clients who have skin that is a little more resistant may require extra treatments to get the same results. For those over 60, whose skin has changed through the aging process and post-menopause hormones, visits twice a week for 6-8 weeks is recommended.

To support the treatments, consistently using a proper skin care line is necessary. Monthly facials and maintenance treatments will greatly improve your success rate. Clients love their results and the slowing of their aging process.

Microcurrent treatments are similar to working out in a gym. If you only take one class or only spend an hour lifting weights, there won't be any improvement in muscle tone. You start going consistently for a month or two and suddenly you have toned muscles. Microcurrent will give you results after one treatment, but in order to achieve long-lasting results, you need to be consistent, like going to the gym. After the initial 6-8 weeks, the treatments will tighten your muscle tone, smooth your wrinkles and lift your sagging skin.

Samantha's Cleanse

I love doing microcurrent treatments because my clients are so satisfied with how their faces feel. In the few months that I have used it with my clients, I have seen noticeable results. The skin tone is more even, and the texture is smooth. Acne, acne scarring and red bumps left after a breakout disappear. Also, the treatment reduces redness, shrinks the capillaries and minimizes the signs of melasma and dark spots on the face. Even the pore size is smaller, leaving the skin feeling softer and smoother. Many of my clients no longer need to wear foundation or heavy face makeup. Instead, their wrinkles are smooth, their face functions without injectables, their sagging skin is tight and they have a jaw line again.

Microcurrent Gels

Gel products are used to help glide the device around the area being treated. My colleague, Shari Rinaldi Braund, created her own gele for estheticians, called Aliven Gele. Shari wanted to fulfill "a need in an esthetician's life." Gels on the market and those provided with the machine contained carbomer components to satisfy the consistency requirements. Rinaldi desired a 'clean product' for her clients. Shari discovered "*many of the gels used are harmful. Carbomer is a cross-link plastic. It is added to a gel in powder form, and the powder can actually become 40% of the actual product, which means it's like sealing plastic on the face.*"[62]

Rinaldi designed the custom gel, Aliven Gele, for estheticians to use with microcurrent treatments. *"It is a lightweight gel that increases the health of our cells and nourishes the skin. Aliven is food for our skin, rather than just a conducting gel. It can also be used as a serum in its own right."*[62] Aliven Gele boosts the hydration level in the skin. I am very satisfied with the product and I enjoy having it for my clients. It is lightweight and has plenty of slip. After a treatment, I can massage the excess into my client's skin because it is nourishing.

If you haven't tried a microcurrent treatment yet and desire to delay the aging process, find an experienced esthetician and schedule an appointment. Microcurrent is a safe, non-invasive facial treatment that can help slow down and reverse signs of aging. It is an effective treatment to prevent and smooth both wrinkles and sagging skin for those in their 20's, 30's, 40's, 50's and up.

AHAS AND BHAS

Alpha Hydroxy Acids (AHAs) and Beta Hydroxy Acids (BHAs) are ingredients that are found in many different skin care lines and products. These two acids are used in spas during facial services and in-home care products.

Alpha Hydroxy Acids

Alpha Hydroxy Acids (AHAs) gained popularity in the 1980's when they generated buzz for reducing wrinkles, decreasing acne and acne scarring and evening skin tone, like melasma. AHAs are used in spas as chemical peels and in products such as cleansers, toners, serums and exfoliants. The most commonly used AHAs are glycolic and lactic acids, but mandelic, malic and tartaric acids are also used. Each AHA has its own origin and benefit to the skin. Chemical peels done in a spa may be a single acid or a blend of two or more AHAs that work to peel the skin while restoring hydration and leaving the skin less irritated. Another reason why peels are blended is so estheticians can combine acids with treatments such as microdermabrasion, laser or injectables.

Source of Alpha Hydroxy Acids

Alpha Hydroxy Acids can be classified as a wounding agent in the skin by the chemistry action on the skin.[63] AHA's have different chemical structures which are organic carboxylic acids with different molecular structures.

The Various Types and Origins of AHA

1) Glycolic acid comes from cane sugar and is the shortest-chain AHA. It works by separating the epidermal cells and can cause erythema (swelling in the skin). This swelling is what has made glycolic acid so popular, because the swelling hides wrinkles, pore size and scarring.

2) Lactic acid comes from sour milk and is the most effective as L-Lactic acid, which is chirally correct. L-Lactic acid is less irritating and an effective tool for dry, acne or discolored skin because it offers hydration, called a "natural moisturizing factor" (NMF) through amino acids. NMF's are known to hold onto water at the skin's surface and the proteins in the skin cells absorb moisture.

3) Mandelic acid comes from bitter almonds and offers both antimicrobial and antiviral properties to the skin. It has a large molecular structure, which means that it is slower to exfoliate the skin without irritation. Mandelic acid is best for clients suffering from acne and melasma. If allergic to almonds, avoid this product.

4) Malic acid comes from apples and berries. It works to promote circulation and reduce capillary size, while softening and gently increasing cell turnover. Malic acid leaves a protective coat on the skin to retain moisture.

5) Tartaric acid comes from grapes, bananas and tamarinds and is the main acid found in wine. Tartaric acid is not widely used in spas or products.

Beta Hydroxy Acids

Beta Hydroxy Acids (BHAs) are best for treating acne because it enters the pores to unglue trapped dirt and oil. BHA's are used at home in acne treatments to keep pores clear of dirt and oil that may lead to acne breakouts. BHAs penetrate the epidermis deeper than an

AHA and provide anti-inflammatory and anti-microbial treatment. *Beta-Hydroxy Acids are recognized as "non-wounding" agents by the chemistry of their action on the skin.*[63] BHA's are oil-soluble and best for treating resistant or clogged pores and blackheads.

Salicyclic Acid

Salicyclic acid is derived from willow bark, which is the main ingredient in aspirin. If a client is allergic to aspirin, BHAs are NOT recommended. It is a carboxylic acid, like AHA's, but has the ability to penetrate the pore and remove impactions (blackheads) and oil-filled follicles.

RETINOLS

Retinols are used for the treatment of acne and aging. These can be prescribed or used in OTC home care products. Retinols are all over the skin care market.

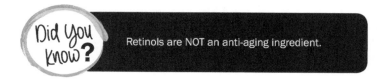

Did you know? Retinols are NOT an anti-aging ingredient.

What is a Retinol?

In 1973, the late renowned dermatologist, Dr. Albert Kligman, MD, PhD, patented the retinoic acid drug, Tretinoin. Vitamin A is still recognized as the single most proven go-to ingredient for improving everything from acne, wrinkles and collagen synthesis to hyperpigmentation.[64] Retinol is a vitamin A derivative and can have a variety of different names, such as retinol, retinoic acid, and retinaldehyde which are the most commonly known. Many people associate retinols with the red, raw, irritated, burning sensation on our skin that we remember from acne days when our dermatologist prescribed it for acne.

While acne was treated with retinol, patients found that it also diminished wrinkles and offered a youthful appearance. This made retinols the hottest anti-aging ingredient to help erase wrinkles. Women are now getting prescriptions for retinol from the dermatologist for this exact reason.

Skin Reactions and Retinols

For those of you who have tried retinols, you know how awful it feels. When first using it, the doctor usually suggests to apply it every other day until you get "used to it." In this time, the skin gets bright red, inflamed, irritated and literally burns. A call to the doctor will garner advice that says "that's normal and to stick with it a few more weeks till your skin gets used to it."

Samantha's Cleanse

From an educated, wellness esthetician and spa owner, your skin reacts in this manner because it is ANGRY! Redness, burning, inflammation and skin irritation is a skin REACTION. Your skin is telling you it doesn't like the product and would like it off your skin. This happens because retinols are extremely irritating and immediately strip the skin. They also peel off several layers of the stratum corneum. The skin has to start fighting and reacts to protect those delicate new skin cells at the dermal/epidermal junction. Without an intact stratum corneum, your skin is unable to protect the dermis from sun damage, irritating at-home ingredients or damage from harsh facial treatments.

Your skin should never feel angry from a product. If it does, you should stop it immediately. Find a licensed esthetician who can calm your skin. She/he can offer products to deliver anti-aging results without suffering skin irritation or inflammation.

Retinaldehyde

Retinaldehyde is a mild version of retinol and is more gentle on the skin. It is beneficial for all skin types, including sensitive skin, acne, rosacea and melasma. Retinaldehyde is vitamin A but our skin converts it to retinoic acid when applied to the skin. A delivery system is key to using retinaldehyde because serums have the carrier ingredients that your skin needs for absorption. If retinaldehyde is encapsulated and is able to penetrate the DEJ, then it will not irritate the skin. It will only irritate the skin if it is left on the skin's surface. There is no benefit to it without the delivery system because it will stay on top of the skin, irritate it and dry it out.

Benefits of Retinaldehyde
- shows anti-microbial effects in the skin which estheticians want to see when treating breakouts
- helps reduce wrinkles by stimulating collagen
- helps to even skin tone by lightening the skin
- works by reducing melanin production in the DEJ, where the melanocytes cells live and are responsible for our skin tone (See Chapter 1)
- decreases the amount of melanin production in our melanocyte cells

Beneficial Vitamin A and the Skin
Not all retinols are bad if they are derived from vitamin A. Our skin needs vitamin A because it converts it into retinoic acid which keeps the skin cells healthy and slows aging by targeting new cells being formed at the DEJ. I use vitamin A serums in my spa and on myself with telling results.

It's the form of vitamin A that irritates the skin. Retinols or any vitamin A product should ONLY be used under the direction of a licensed professional or physician. Salespeople do not know the difference between the stability versus instability of an ingredient and they are not trained to understand skin. *To overcome irritation and stability issues, retinol chemists have also used specialized delivery forms that encapsulate active retinol in a polymer stream to slowly "feed" the skin a more stable, bioactive form with minimal irritation.*[64] By encapsulating the retinols, they release more slowly than when

208 | Skin Deep

you directly apply them to the skin. Encapsulation allows the retinols to get to the dermal/epidermal junction to repair DNA damage and restore health to the new cells as they are born.

Now that you are familiar with the role an esthetician has in your life and the various and most common services available, take the next step for your skin health. Find an esthetician that will plan goals with you to help your skin look and feel its best.

TIPS TO FINDING A GOOD ESTHETICIAN:

- Ask your friends or find a moms group on Facebook who can recommend an esthetician.
- Research online – website, social media, review sites to see if you like their work.
- Call or schedule a consultation. Most estheticians offer free consultations.
- Bring all your current skin care products and ask questions during the consultation that specifically relate to your skin concerns.
- Some estheticians may offer a mini facial to see how your skin responds.
- If you feel great energy and love her touch, then schedule a facial. If not, move on to the next esthetician until you find the one that resonates the best with YOU!
- You and your esthetician are going to build a partnership and friendship over the next several decades. You want to find someone you click with and you can trust with your skin.

Chapter 11:
Rules to Live By

The beauty industry is flooded with skin care products and misinformation about which products to use. Manufacturers label products to entice us to purchase them with certain key words. Estheticians are highly trained and very well-versed in the skin. We touch our clients on a daily basis and we get to know the skin by feeling it and can learn a lot by putting our hands on your beautiful face. We are required by state board law to get continuing education classes to keep our licenses current and many of these classes are about the science of the skin. We are continuing to learn how to better serve our clients and keep current with the latest trends in modalities and ingredients. All the estheticians I know don't just get the bare minimum to keep their licenses up. They go above and beyond. They are hungry and eager for knowledge about the skin. Skin is our passion and we enjoy helping our clients' skin look and feel better as we continue to age.

This section is dedicated to Lori Crete. I am extremely grateful to Lori for being my mentor who has helped me grow as a business owner, as an esthetician and has helped me develop the culture of my spa.

I've enlisted the help of Lori, licensed esthetician, spa owner, president and founder of The Esthetician Mentor.[60] Crete helps clarify misinformation and how best to purchase skin care products. Buying online to save money is not always beneficial for your skin or your wallet.

ESTHETICIANS ARE PROFESSIONALS EDUCATED IN SKIN CARE

When Lori Crete meets her clients, she tells them "I want to be your skin care guru. Please call me anytime for advice about your skin and I will help you pick your products. I want to make sure you have products that are customized for your specific need. There is no need to play the expensive and time-consuming 'which product is right for me' game."[60]

All really good licensed estheticians have this same approach. When I was starting my business, Lori encouraged me to be a professional who is an expert in helping people understand the importance of the correct products for their specific needs. It is not about 'selling' product; it's about helping our clients get what they need to meet their skin care goals.

Estheticians are extremely important when it comes to making skin care purchases. We have the knowledge, expertise and hands-on experience to understand skin reactions, what it needs to stay healthy and how to slow down the aging process. Trusted estheticians get to know your skin. A customized skincare program will end up saving you money and skin problems in the long-term. Estheticians ARE the experts.

LET US SPOIL YOU

Our time spent with you is quality time, and we need every minute that is scheduled to properly give you the services you require. We also want to give you your money's worth. In a spa, time is of the essence, and our schedules are tight. To serve all our clients, we need to work on an extremely tight schedule. When people run late, cancel at the last minute or don't show at all, it shifts our entire day. Unfortunately, that impacts the person who is late and the people after them. The session may have to be cut short which means the entire process was not applied. Missed or late appointments cause stress in an environment that is supposed to be serene. We love what we do, and we want to give each client the same level of service, make it enjoyable and lead your skin to better health. Please be the on-time, courteous client so we can spoil you with highest level of care.

IMPORTANCE OF AN ESTHETICIAN WHEN MAKING SKINCARE PURCHASES

Estheticians offer you products that will make your skin look and feel best, no matter the season or skin condition. Estheticians offer top-quality, professional skincare products made in smaller batches, that use delivery systems to get the product to target the new cells being born. Professional quality products are more beneficial to the skin with less irritation and better results.

There is no need to keep searching for that perfect product and wasting money on products that do not work for your skin. When a friend or co-worker talks you into buying a product that works for her skin, I don't recommend going out and buying it. It might not work for your skin, because you have different skin types and needs; what works for your friend will not work for you.

WHY BUYING ONLINE WON'T SAVE YOUR MONEY

Buying anything online is super easy and saves us time and money, right? Beware when buying skin care products online. They are not regulated, and there is a chance you will receive a used product or a product that you did not order.

Samantha's Story Time

Katt Philipps is a licensed esthetician, owner of Grafin Skin & Beauty and Petal & Herb. In her blog, she shared an unpleasant client experience. *"After purchasing her lash enhancing serum online for the significant discount, she came in to see me. Her lashes fell out in clumps! She trusted the online retailer for her purchase and received a counterfeit."* [65]

This is so scary. Unfortunately, it is not the first time I've heard stories from estheticians about their clients purchasing the wrong products, believing they are getting quality at a lower price.

This incident could have been far worse; the lash product had the potential to permanently damage her vision. Currently, it is hard to tell if her client's lashes will grow back due to damage of the hair follicle, but they are hopeful for a full recovery in 3-6 months!

THE RESALE

Websites provide the perfect platform for those who are looking to make a quick buck. Many stories arise out of these situations, and oftentimes at the expense of our own health. For example: An esthetician, wants to bring in a new line without losing money on the current stock. The rep from the new skincare line buys the remaining stock. She didn't ask for expiration dates, nor did she look to see if any of it was used. The rep now has an opportunity to sell it online for a discount.

The customer is searching online for the usual serum and sees it at a great discount. Buys it, uses it. It kind of smells funny, but that's okay. Customer uses it, it irritates her skin. She can't figure out why the skin changed and she tries to send it back. The company may not accept returns, or may send a replacement, which is worse than the first. Unfortunately, this is a very common scenario, and I hear stories all the time from clients and other esthetician's clients.

DAMAGED GOODS

We are familiar with beauty stores that sell every line created for hair, skin, makeup and nails. Some even have a salon or spa attached to the retail store. They have shelves upon shelves of products. Oftentimes, the products expire and should be tossed. Sometimes the product arrives damaged or tampered, and they toss it into the dumpster out back. There are actually people that dumpster dive outside these stores or department stores to steal the products and sell them online. If the product looks damaged or tampered, they just repackage it and sell online for a discount. That serum just purchased can be expired, in a new bottle or may not be the same product the consumer expected. It may be a different product or mixture of several products. This is dangerous and harmful for both the skin and body. Be sure you know where the products originated.

Crete explains, *"Internet shopping is not going away. This is why having an open communication with your esthetician is so important."*[60] When you buy from your esthetician, you will not get an expired or damaged product. Estheticians buy their products directly from the company, and those products are made in small batches. Crete says, *"Find an esthetician who will ship products directly to you or ask if they have an online store."*[60] Many professional skincare companies are aware of online purchasing and have shut down those who are selling their products under a different company name. The skincare line I offer at my spa has a zero-tolerance rule, and I follow their rules when selling or shipping products. This is very important because the company wants to ensure every client receives the expected product for their healthy skin care regimen.

BE PREPARED AND BE COMPLETELY COMFORTABLE

When seeing your esthetician for the first time, come prepared with your current products, questions and skin issues. The spa is a safe and confidential space. If you have it, we have heard it all and seen it all. Take comfort in knowing that we are trustworthy, compassionate and non-judgmental. We are here for you to have a wonderful experience

214 | Skin Deep

and for you to feel beautiful on the inside and out. Keep the lines of communication open, and you will receive the greatest benefits we can offer.

There you have it, all the tools, tips and trade secrets, which officially makes YOU an educated consumer! Congratulations on putting in the time to educate yourself on why skin care is so important and why it should be important to you. After all, your skin is the organ that we look at first. Why not treat your skin with the love and respect it deserves?

Here's to loving the skin you're in!

XO,
Samantha

References

1   MedicineNet.com. Definition of Dermis. http://www.medicinenet.com/
    script/main/art.asp?articlekey=2958

2   National Center for Biotechnology Information, U.S. National Library of
    Medicine. *"Challenges and opportunities in dermal/transdermal delivery."*
    http://www.ncbi.nlm.nih.gov/pmc/articles/PMC2995530/

3   Ronert, Marc A. *"How Delivery Systems Change Skin Care Effectiveness."*
    Skin Inc. Magazine http://www.skininc.com/skinscience/physiology/
    How-Delivery-Systems-Change-Skin-Care-Effectiveness-261313781.html

4   The Doctors via Rajauria, Arpit. *"What it Looks Like When You Don't
    Wash Off Your Makeup for a Month."* https://youtube/eKb2A5fxiUE

5   Scheve, Tom. *"What is in Sweat?"* How Stuff Works. http://health.
    howstuffworks.com/wellness/men/sweating-odor/what-is-in-sweat.htm

6   Manzo, Robert. *"Ingredient Labels Explained."* Skin Inc. Magazine.
    http://www.skininc.com/skinscience/ingredients/Ingredient-Labels-
    Explained-209186181.html

7   Medscape Medical News. *"Oncology – Link Between Parabens and
    Breast Cancer?"* http://www.medscape.com/viewarticle/757561#vp_3
    *Fall, 2016, this page was unexpectedly converted to a membership site,
    documentation is within site.

8   Personal Care Products Council On-line Infobase.
     Cosmetic Ingredient Review Expert Panel 2010 http://online.
     personalcarecouncil.org/ctfa-static/online/lists/cir-pdfs/FR548.pdf

9   Szalay, Jessie. "Inflammation: Causes, Symptoms and Anti-Inflammatory
     Diet." LiveScience. http://www.livescience.com/52344-inflammation.html

10   Uribarri, Jaime., et al. "Advanced Glycation End Products in Foods
     and a Practical Guide to Their Reduction in the Diet." *US National
     Library of Medicine: National Institutes of Health.* http://www.ncbi.nlm.
     nih.gov/pmc/articles/PMC3704564/

11   Ware, Megan, RDN, LD. "Ginger: Health Benefits, Facts, Research."
     Medical News Today. http://www.medicalnewstoday.com/
     articles/265990.php

12   The World's Healthiest Foods. "What's New and Beneficial
     About Turmeric?" http://www.whfoods.com/genpage.
     php?tname=foodspice&dbid=78

13   Dumas, Kiley. "5 Health Benefits of Avocados." *Full Circle.* http://www.
     fullcircle.com/goodfoodlife/2012/06/21/5-health-benefits-of-avocados/

14   MDHealth.com. "Cold Water Fish." *MD Health.* http://www.md-health.
     com/Cold-Water-Fish.html

15   Lima, Cristiano. "57 Names of Sugar." *Prevention Magazine.* http://
     www.prevention.com/food/healthy-eating-tips/the-57-names-of-sugar/
     yellow-sugar

16   Wikipedia. "Candida." https://en.wikipedia.org/wiki/Candida_(fungus)

17   Pontillo, Rachael. "10 Things About the Immune System." *Dermascope.*
     http://www.dermascope.com/wellness/10-things-about-the-immune-sys
     tem?highlight=WyJjYW5kaWRhIl0=#.VshNV2A-CLI

18   Richards, Lisa. "6 Easy Steps to Kick Your Sugar Cravings."
     The Candida Diet. http://www.thecandidadiet.com/6-easy-tips-to-kick-
     your-sugar-cravings/

19   Montaguge-King, Danne. "Myths and Realities of Acne." *Dermascope.*

http://www.dermascope.com/acne/myths-and-realities-of-acne?highligh
t=WyJnbHV0ZW4iXQ==#.VshY_mA-CLI

20   Gluten Free Society. "Guidelines for Avoiding Gluten." https://www.
     glutenfreesociety.org/guidelines-for-avoiding-gluten-unsafe-ingredients-
     for-gluten-sensitivity/

21   Kids With Food Allergies. "Frequently Asked Questions about the
     Food Allergen Labeling Consumer Act (FALCPA)" http://www.
     kidswithfoodallergies.org/page/label-law-food-allergen-labeling-
     consumer-protection-act.aspx

22   Ede, Georgia, M.D. "Dairy." *Diagnosis Diet.* http://www.diagnosisdiet.
     com/food/dairy/

23   Wikipedia. "Casein." *Wikipedia.* https://en.wikipedia.org/wiki/Casein

24   "What is Lactose Intolerance?" *No Whey.* http://www.nowhey.org/
     aboutli.htm

25   "Stress Symptoms, Signs and Causes." HelpGuide. http://www.helpguide.
     org/articles/stress/stress-symptoms-causes-and-effects.htm

26   Staff, Mayo Clinic. "Stress Symptoms: Effects on Your Body and
     Behavior." *Mayo Clinic.* http://www.mayoclinic.org/healthy-lifestyle/
     stress-management/in-depth/stress-symptoms/art-20050987

27   Ferrill, Erin. "Dry vs. Dehydration: Causes and Symptoms." *Skin Inc
     Magazine.* http://www.skininc.com/skinscience/physiology/Dry-vs-
     Dehydrated-Skin-Causes-and-Treatments-261315311.html

28   Stress Management Health Centre. "Effects of Stress on Your Body."
     WebMD. http://www.webmd.boots.com/stress-management/physical-
     stress-symptoms

29   "Circadian Rhythms Facts Sheet." *National Institute of General Medical
     Sciences.* https://www.nigms.nih.gov/Education/Pages/Factsheet_
     CircadianRhythms.aspx

30   Sleep Association.org "What is Sleep?" *American Sleep Association.*
     https://www.sleepassociation.org/patients-general-public/what-is-sleep/

31   Harvard Health Publications. "Blue Light has a Dark Side." *Harvard Medical School*. http://www.health.harvard.edu/staying-healthy/blue-light-has-a-dark-side

32   Sleep Medicine. "Green Light Affects Circadian Rhythm" *Division of Harvard Medical School*. https://sleep.med.harvard.edu/news/356/Green+Light+Affects+Circadian+Rhythm

33   Staff, Mayo Clinic. "Exercise: 7 Benefits of Regular Physical Activity." *Mayo Clinic*. http://www.mayoclinic.org/healthy-lifestyle/fitness/in-depth/exercise/art-20048389

34   Sjoberg,Valerie. "Functional Medicine: What's All the Hype?" *The Chopra Center*. http://www.chopra.com/articles/functional-medicine-what%E2%80%99s-all-the-hype

35   "Core Principles of Functional Medicine." *The Institute for Functional Medicine*. https://www.functionalmedicine.org/files/library/six-core-principles.pdf

36   Alternet- The Cosmetics Racket: Why the Beauty industry can get away with charging a fortune for makeup - http://www.alternet.org/story/148140/the_cosmetics_racket%3A_why_the_beauty_industry_can_get_away_with_charging_a_fortune_for_makeup

37   Thomasnet.com: Cosmetic Manufacturing Chemist, Inc - http://www.thomasnet.com/capabilities-services.html?heading=55610646&WTZO=Recently+Viewed+Supplier&cid=30560508&WTZO=See+More+Capabilities+Services

38   Johnson, Ben, M.D. President, Founder and Formulator of Osmosis Skin Care. Interview, 2016. www.osmosisskincare.com

39   Written Work. "Louis Pasteur and the Discovery of Molecular Chirality." *Conf.Gal*. http://www.ufr926.upmc.fr/totem_g/seminaires/GAL.pdf

40   Dermascope Magazine. "Chirally Correct Skin Care…or is it?" *Dermascope*. http://www.dermascope.com/chemistry/chirally-correct-skin-care-or-is-it#.VyF9QbQ-Bok

41   Löffler H, Happle R. "Profile of irritant patch testing with detergents:

sodium lauryl sulfate, sodium laureth sulfate and alkyl polyglucoside."
US National Library of Medicine: National Institutes of Health.
http://www.ncbi.nlm.nih.gov/pubmed/12641575

42 Polla, Ada & Pouillot, Anne. 2012 "Controversial Ingredients: Setting
the Record Straight." *Skin Inc Magazine.* http://www.skininc.com/
skinscience/ingredients/138355864.html

43 Personal Care Products Council On-line Infobase. *Cosmetic Ingredient
Review Expert Panel 2010 (DEA)* http://online.personalcarecouncil.org/
ctfa-static/online/lists/cir-pdfs/FR575.pdf and www.cir-safety.org - type
in Diethanolamine to access "Final Report"

44 Personal Care Products Council On-line Infobase. *Cosmetic Ingredient
Review Expert Panel 2010 (MEA)* http://online.personalcarecouncil.org/
ctfa-static/online/lists/cir-pdfs/FR604.pdf

45 Personal Care Products Council On-line Infobase. *Cosmetic Ingredient
Review Expert Panel 2010 (TEA)* http://online.personalcarecouncil.org/
ctfa-static/online/lists/cir-pdfs/pr594.pdf

46 Personal Care Products Council On-line Infobase. *Cosmetic Ingredient
Review Expert Panel 2010 (Sodium Hydroxide)* http://online.
personalcarecouncil.org/ctfa-static/online/lists/cir-pdfs/FR703.pdf

47 Personal Care Products Council On-line Infobase. *Cosmetic Ingredient
Review Expert Panel 2010 (Triclosan)* http://online.personalcarecouncil.
org/ctfa-static/online/lists/cir-pdfs/FR569.pdf

48 Personal Care Products Council On-line Infobase. *Cosmetic Ingredient
Review Expert Panel 2010: Annual Review of Cosmetic Ingredient Safety
Assessments. 2005/2006.* http://online.personalcarecouncil.org/ctfa-
static/online/lists/cir-pdfs/prn547.PDF

49 American Cancer Society. "Antiperspirants and Breast Cancer Risk: The
Claims." http://www.cancer.org/cancer/cancercauses/othercarcinogens/
athome/antiperspirants-and-breast-cancer-risk

50 Written Report. "Final Report of the Safety Assessment of Alcohol
Denat..." *International Journal of Toxicology.* http://online.
personalcarecouncil.org/ctfa-static/online/lists/cir-pdfs/PR273.PDF

51   U.S. Food & Drug Administration, U.S. Department of Health & Human Services. "Color Additives and Cosmetics." http://www.fda. gov/ForIndustry/ColorAdditives/ColorAdditivesinSpecificProducts/ InCosmetics/ucm110032.htm

52   Electronic Code of Federal Regulations, Part 74, U.S. Government Publishing Office. *"Listing of Color Additives Subject to Certification."* http://www.ecfr.gov/cgi-bin/retrieveECFR?gp=&SID=17723345ba7c363ef 25a68e9776aa2cd&r=PART&n=21y1.0.1.1.28#se21.1.74_12052

53   U.S. Food & Drug Administration, U.S. Department of Health & Human Services. "Fragrances in Cosmetics." http://www.fda.gov/cosmetics/ productsingredients/ingredients/ucm388821.htm

54   U.S. Food & Drug Administration, U.S. Department of Health & Human Services. "Phthalates." http://www.fda.gov/Cosmetics/ ProductsIngredients/Ingredients/ucm128250.htm

55   National Service Center for Environmental Publications, United States Environmental Protection Agency. "Exposure And Risk Assessment For Phthalate Esters" *(page 73 section 3-10), (page 81 section 3-18), (page 89 section 5-7), (page 103 section 7-11),* http://nepis.epa.gov/Exe/ ZyNET.exe/2000M00O.txt?ZyActionD=ZyDocument&Client=EPA&Ind ex=1981%20Thru%201985&Docs=&Query=&Time=&EndTime=&Search Method=1&TocRestrict=n&Toc=&TocEntry=&QField=&QFieldYear=&Q FieldMonth=&QFieldDay=&UseQField=&IntQFieldOp=0&ExtQFieldOp= 0&XmlQuery=&File=D%3A%5CZYFILES%5CINDEX%20DATA%5C81T HRU85%5CTXT%5C00000005%5C2000M00O.txt&User=ANONYMOUS &Password=anonymous&SortMethod=h%7C-&MaximumDocuments=1& FuzzyDegree=0&ImageQuality=r75g8/r75g8/x150y150g16/i425&Display= p%7Cf&DefSeekPage=x&SearchBack=ZyActionL&Back=ZyActionS&Back Desc=Results%20page&MaximumPages=1&ZyEntry=22

56   U.S. Food & Drug Administration, U.S. Department of Health & Human Services. "Parabens in Cosmetics." http://www.fda.gov/cosmetics/ productsingredients/ingredients/ucm128042.htm

57   U.S. Food & Drug Administration. "Summary of Color Additives for Use in the US in Foods, Drugs, Cosmetics, and Medical Devices." *U.S. Department of Health & Human Services.* http://www.fda.gov/ ForIndustry/ColorAdditives/ColorAdditiveInventories/ucm115641.htm

58   CA.gov. OEHHA Science for a Healthy California. "Proposition 65."
      http://oehha.ca.gov/prop65.html

59   Major, Abbie. Licensed Esthetician, Spa Owner of Abbie Major Skin
      Love. Interview, 2016. www.abbiemajor.com

60   Crete, Lori. Licensed Esthetician, Spa Owner of The Spa 10, Author, and
      President of The Esthetician Mentor. Interview, 2016. www.thespa10.com
      and www.theestheticianmentor.com

61   Rochman, Chelsea M. "Scientific Evidence Supports a Ban on Microbeads."
      Environmental Science & Technology. http://pubs.acs.org/doi/
      pdfplus/10.1021/acs.est.5b03909

62   Rinaldi Braund, Shari. Licensed Esthetician, Spa Owner of Skin Caring
      by Shari and Creator of Aliven Gele. Interview, 2016.
      www.skincaringservices.com

63   Dermascope Magazine. "Understanding Acids." *Dermascope.* http://www.
      dermascope.com/chemistry/understanding-acids?highlight=WyJnbHljb2xp
      YyIsImFjaWQiLCJnbHljb2xpYyBhY2lkIl0=#.VycwNbQ-CLI

64   Dhatt, Dr. Sam. "Vitamin A: New Applications and Outcomes." *Skin Inc
      Magazine.* http://www.skininc.com/skinscience/ingredients/Vitamin-A-
      New-Applications-and-Outcomes-200633731.html

65   Phillip, Katt. Licensed Ethetician, Spa Owner of Grafin Skin & Beauty
      and Owner of Petal & Herb and Blogger. "Amazon: Counterfeit Cosmetic
      Danger." http://blog.grafinskinandbeauty.com/counterfeit-cosmetic-
      danger/